Table of Contents

Introduction

- Welcome Message
- Importance of Nutrition During Pregnancy
- How to Use This Cookbook

Section 1: First Trimester

Understanding the First Trimester

Nutrition Guidelines for the First Trimester

Essential Nutrients and Their Functions

Foods to Embrace and Avoid

First Trimester Meal Planning Tips

Recipes for the First Trimester

- Energizing Breakfasts
- Comforting Soups and Stews
- Nourishing Snack Ideas
- Satisfying Main Courses
- Rejuvenating Beverages and Smoothies

Extra Tips and Advice

- Coping with Morning Sickness
- Handling Food Aversions and Cravings
- Safe Exercise and Physical Activity

Section 2: Second Trimester

- Understanding the Second Trimester
- Nutrition Guidelines for the Second Trimester
- Growth and Development Milestones

- Iron-Rich Foods for Blood Support
- Second Trimester Meal Planning Strategies

Recipes for the Second Trimester

- Power-Packed Salads and Bowls
- Wholesome Pasta and Grain Dishes
- Healthy Desserts and Treats
- Hydrating Infusions and Drinks

Extra Tips and Advice

- Managing Heartburn and Indigestion
- Maintaining a Balanced Diet
- Preparing for Labor and Delivery

Section 3: Third Trimester

- Understanding the Third Trimester
- Nutrition Guidelines for the Third Trimester
- Final Preparations for Birth and Beyond
- Calcium-Rich Foods for Bone Development
- Third Trimester Meal Planning Techniques

Recipes for the Third Trimester

- Nutrient-Dense Smoothie Bowls
- Comforting One-Pot Meals
- Energy-Boosting Snacks
- Soothing Herbal Teas and Elixirs

Extra Tips and Advice

- Dealing with Swelling and Discomfort
- Preparing for Breastfeeding
- Creating a Relaxing Birth Environment

Section 4: Postpartum and Beyond

- Postpartum Nutrition and Recovery
- Breastfeeding Diet Essentials
- Quick and Healthy Meals for New Moms
- Introducing Solids to Your Baby
- Continuing Healthy Eating Habits

Recipes for Postpartum and Beyond

- Quick and Nutritious Breakfast Ideas
- Easy-to-Prepare Lunches and Dinners
- Snacks for New Moms and Babies
- Homemade Baby Food Recipes

Extra Tips and Advice

- Self-Care for New Moms
- Bonding Activities with Your Baby
- Long-Term Nutritional Guidelines

Conclusion

- Recap of Key Points
- Encouragement and Final Words

Introduction

- Welcome Message
- Importance of Nutrition During Pregnancy
- How to Use This Cookbook

Welcome to the Pregnancy Cookbook by Trimester: Nutritious and Healthy Recipes for a Healthy 9 Months, Guides for You and Your Developing Baby and Beyond!

Congratulations on this exciting journey towards motherhood. This cookbook is designed to be your faithful companion, providing a wealth of information and delectable recipes tailored to support you throughout the miraculous journey of pregnancy.

Pregnancy is a remarkable phase filled with changes and anticipation. It's a time when your body undergoes incredible transformations to nurture and support the growth of a new life within. As such, the significance of proper nutrition during pregnancy cannot be overstated. What you eat plays a crucial role in not just your health but also in the development and well-being of your baby.

The nutrients you consume during these nine months have a direct impact on your baby's growth, brain development, and overall health. A well-balanced diet enriched with essential vitamins, minerals, proteins, and healthy fats is fundamental to ensure both you and your baby receive the necessary nourishment.

Understanding the importance of a balanced diet, this cookbook has been meticulously crafted to guide you through each trimester, offering recipes that cater to the specific nutritional needs during different stages of pregnancy. Whether you're dealing with morning sickness in the first trimester, experiencing heightened energy needs in the second trimester, or focusing on optimal fetal development in the third trimester, this cookbook aims to provide recipes that are both delicious and nutritionally dense.

Moreover, this cookbook goes beyond just recipes. It includes comprehensive guides and information tailored to support you at every step. From nutritional guides outlining key nutrients required during pregnancy to practical tips on meal planning, managing cravings, and even postpartum nutrition, this cookbook is a holistic resource to assist you throughout this incredible journey.

Our aim is not just to offer delectable recipes but to empower you with knowledge and tools that will help you make informed and healthy choices for yourself and your growing baby. We believe that by nourishing yourself with wholesome, nutritious meals, you're not only promoting your own well-being but also laying a strong foundation for your baby's health and development.

So, dive into these pages, explore the recipes, and embark on this culinary adventure designed to make your pregnancy journey as healthy, vibrant, and joyous as possible. Here's to a journey filled with delicious meals, good health, and the anticipation of welcoming a new life into this world. Enjoy the journey, savor the flavors, and cherish every moment of this remarkable experience.

Section 1

First Trimester

- **Understanding the First Trimester**

From conception to around week 12, the first trimester of pregnancy is an important and life-changing time. The developing baby and the mother's body are going through a tremendous period of change and development. To comprehend the first trimester, one must explore the developmental, emotional, and physiological features that make up this first trimester of pregnancy.

Physical Changes

From the moment of conception, the female body begins a series of remarkable changes. One of the earliest signs is a missed period, which often prompts a woman to take a pregnancy test. Hormonal shifts, particularly the increased production of human chorionic gonadotropin (hCG) and progesterone, are responsible for various physical changes during this phase.

Common physical symptoms experienced in the first trimester include:

- *Morning sickness:* Nausea and vomiting, which can occur at any time of the day.
- Fatigue: Due to increased hormonal levels and the body's energy being directed towards fetal development.
- *Breast tenderness:* Hormonal changes can lead to breast soreness and enlargement.
- *Frequent urination:* As the uterus expands, it puts pressure on the bladder.
- *Food aversions and cravings:* Changes in taste preferences influenced by hormonal fluctuations.
- *Increased vaginal discharge:* A normal response to hormonal changes but should be monitored for any abnormalities.

Fetal Development

During the first trimester, the embryo undergoes rapid development. At around five to six weeks, the embryo's heart begins to beat, and basic structures such as the brain, spinal cord, and limbs start forming. By the end of the first trimester, the fetus has recognizable human features, with all major organs and systems in place.

Notable milestones during this period include:

- *Weeks 4-5:* Neural tube formation, which eventually develops into the brain and spinal cord.
- *Weeks 6-7:* Heartbeat becomes detectable, and facial features begin to form.
- *Weeks 8-10:* Limb buds develop into arms and legs, and the fetus starts moving, although it's not felt by the mother yet.
- *Weeks 11-12:* Fetus grows rapidly, and external genitalia begin to differentiate, although it might not be visible on ultrasound.

Emotional and Mental Well-being

The first trimester can be a rollercoaster of emotions for expectant mothers. Mixed feelings of excitement, anxiety, and mood swings are common and attributed to hormonal fluctuations and the anticipation of impending changes.

Many women experience worries about miscarriage during this period due to the highest risk being within the first trimester. This concern can significantly impact mental health. It's crucial for mothers to seek support from their partners, family, friends, or healthcare professionals to manage stress and anxiety.

Additionally, establishing a healthy routine that includes proper nutrition, regular prenatal check-ups, moderate exercise, and adequate rest is essential for both the physical and mental well-being of the mother and the developing fetus.

In conclusion, the first trimester is a critical phase in pregnancy, marked by profound physical, emotional, and developmental changes. Understanding these changes is crucial for expectant mothers to navigate this period with knowledge, care, and support, setting the foundation for a healthy pregnancy and the well-being of both mother and child.

- **Nutrition Guidelines for the First Trimester**

During the first trimester of pregnancy, proper nutrition is crucial as it sets the foundation for the baby's growth and development. While the initial months may bring about nausea, vomiting, and food aversions for many women, maintaining a healthy diet remains essential to support both the mother and the growing fetus.

Folic Acid and Vitamins

- Begin by taking prenatal vitamins or supplements prescribed by your healthcare provider before conception and throughout the first trimester. Folic acid is especially vital in the early stages of pregnancy as it helps prevent neural tube defects in the baby.
- Ensure you're getting adequate amounts of other essential vitamins like vitamin D, vitamin C, and iron, either through diet or supplements.

Hydration

- Drink plenty of water to stay hydrated. Aim for at least 8-10 glasses of water per day. Dehydration can lead to complications, so maintaining fluid intake is crucial.

Balanced Diet

- Consume a well-balanced diet that includes a variety of nutrients. Opt for whole foods such as fruits, vegetables, lean proteins, whole grains, and dairy products.
- Focus on incorporating foods rich in folate, such as leafy greens, legumes, citrus fruits, and fortified grains, to support the baby's neural development.

Foods to Avoid

- Steer clear of certain foods that can pose a risk during pregnancy. Avoid raw or undercooked meats, unpasteurized dairy products, and fish high in mercury. Also, limit caffeine intake.

Small, Frequent Meals

- To manage nausea and morning sickness, try eating smaller, more frequent meals throughout the day rather than large meals. Opt for easily digestible foods like crackers, toast, or ginger tea to help alleviate nausea.

Listen to Your Body

- Respect your body's signals and cravings. If certain foods make you feel queasy, try finding alternatives that provide similar nutrients. Additionally, if you're experiencing
- severe symptoms like hyperemesis gravidarum (severe nausea and vomiting), seek medical advice.

Healthy Snacking

- Keep healthy snacks readily available. Snack on fruits, nuts, yogurt, or whole-grain crackers to curb hunger and maintain stable blood sugar levels.

Avoid Alcohol and Smoking

- Completely avoid alcohol and smoking during pregnancy. Both can have severe detrimental effects on the baby's development.

Consult Healthcare Provider

- Regularly consult with your healthcare provider to ensure you're meeting your nutritional needs. They may recommend specific dietary adjustments based on your individual health status and needs.

Rest and Relaxation

Don't overlook the importance of rest and relaxation. Fatigue is common during the first trimester due to hormonal changes, so ensure you get adequate rest and sleep.

Remember, every pregnancy is unique, and these guidelines should be personalized based on individual health factors and recommendations from your healthcare provider. By focusing on a nutrient-rich diet and making healthy lifestyle choices, you'll be supporting the optimal development of your baby during this crucial phase of pregnancy.

- **Essential Nutrients and Their Functions**

Absolutely! During the first trimester of pregnancy, proper nutrition plays a crucial role in supporting the growth and development of the fetus. Here are some essential nutrients and their functions that are particularly vital during this phase:

Folic Acid (Folate):

- *Function:* Folate is fundamental for preventing neural tube defects in the developing fetus, particularly during the first few weeks of pregnancy when the neural tube is forming.
- *Sources:* Leafy green vegetables, fortified cereals, legumes, and supplements recommended by healthcare providers.

Iron:

- *Function:* Iron is essential for producing red blood cells, aiding in the delivery of oxygen to both the mother and the growing baby. It's crucial in preventing anemia during pregnancy.
- *Sources:* Red meat, poultry, fish, fortified cereals, beans, and spinach.

Calcium:

- *Function:* Calcium is necessary for the development of strong bones and teeth in the baby. It also helps with nerve signaling, muscle function, and blood clotting.
- *Sources:* Dairy products, leafy greens, fortified plant-based milk, and supplements if needed.

Omega-3 Fatty Acids:

- *Function:* Omega-3s, especially DHA (docosahexaenoic acid), support the baby's brain and eye development.
- *Sources:* Fatty fish (like salmon and sardines), flaxseeds, chia seeds, walnuts, and prenatal supplements.

Protein:

- *Function:* Proteins are the building blocks for the baby's growth, contributing to the development of tissues and organs.
- *Sources:* Lean meats, poultry, fish, dairy products, legumes, nuts, and seeds.

Vitamin D:

- *Function:* Vitamin D aids in the absorption of calcium, promoting healthy bone development in the fetus.
- *Sources:* Sun exposure (limited), fortified dairy or plant-based products, and supplements if recommended.

Vitamin C:

- *Function:* Vitamin C boosts the immune system, aids in the absorption of iron, and assists in tissue repair and growth.
- *Sources:* Citrus fruits, berries, bell peppers, tomatoes, and broccoli.

Zinc:

- *Function:* Zinc supports the immune system, aids in cell division and growth, and helps in the development of the baby's organs.
- *Sources:* Meats, dairy, nuts, whole grains, and legumes.

Iodine:

- *Function:* Iodine is crucial for the baby's brain and nervous system development.
- *Sources:* Iodized salt, seafood, dairy products, and some bread.

Vitamin B6:

- *Function:* Vitamin B6 helps in the formation of red blood cells and supports the baby's brain development.
- *Sources:* Poultry, fish, bananas, fortified cereals, and potatoes.

During the first trimester, it's common for pregnant individuals to experience morning sickness or nausea, which might impact their ability to consume certain foods. Prenatal supplements can be beneficial to fill in nutritional gaps, but it's always best to consult with a healthcare professional for personalized advice. Eating a varied and balanced diet, rich in these essential nutrients, is pivotal for a healthy pregnancy and baby during the first trimester and beyond.

- **Foods to Embrace and Avoid**

During the first trimester of pregnancy, a woman's body undergoes significant changes to support the growth and development of the baby. Proper nutrition during this period is crucial for the health of both the mother and the developing fetus. Here's a comprehensive guide to foods to embrace and avoid during the first trimester.

- **Foods to Embrace:**

1. *Folate-rich Foods:* Folate is crucial in preventing neural tube defects in the baby. Embrace leafy greens like spinach, broccoli, citrus fruits, beans, and fortified cereals.

2. *Lean Proteins:* Incorporate lean meats, poultry, fish, eggs, and plant-based protein sources like lentils and beans. They provide essential amino acids necessary for fetal growth.

3. *Dairy Products:* Calcium is vital for bone development. Opt for milk, cheese, yogurt, and fortified plant-based alternatives to meet calcium needs.

4. *Whole Grains:* Complex carbohydrates from whole grains like brown rice, quinoa, whole wheat bread, and oats provide sustained energy and essential nutrients like fiber.

5. *Healthy Fats:* Omega-3 fatty acids are crucial for the baby's brain and eye development. Consume sources like salmon, chia seeds, flaxseeds, and walnuts.

6. *Fruits and Vegetables:* Colorful fruits and veggies provide an array of vitamins, minerals, and antioxidants. Aim for a variety to ensure a wide range of nutrients.

7. *Hydration:* Drink plenty of water throughout the day to support blood volume expansion, aid digestion, and maintain amniotic fluid levels.

- **Foods to Avoid:**

1. *High-Mercury Fish:* Certain fish like shark, swordfish, king mackerel, and tilefish contain high levels of mercury that can harm the developing nervous system of the fetus.

2. *Raw or Undercooked Meats:* To prevent foodborne illnesses, avoid undercooked or raw meats and poultry as they may contain harmful bacteria like salmonella or toxoplasma.

3. *Unpasteurized Dairy Products:* These can harbor harmful bacteria like listeria, which can lead to infections. Stick to pasteurized options for safety.

4. *Excessive Caffeine:* High caffeine intake has been associated with an increased risk of miscarriage. Limit caffeine consumption to around 200mg per day.

5. *Raw Sprouts:* Avoid raw sprouts like alfalfa, clover, or radish as they may carry bacteria and pose a risk of foodborne illness.

6. *Certain Herbal Teas and Supplements:* Some herbs can have adverse effects on pregnancy. Consult a healthcare provider before consuming herbal teas or supplements.

7. *Alcohol and Smoking:* Completely avoid alcohol and smoking during pregnancy as they can lead to severe birth defects and developmental issues.

Always consult with a healthcare provider or a registered dietitian for personalized guidance on nutrition during pregnancy. These guidelines can help support a healthy and safe first trimester, providing the essential nutrients needed for the baby's growth while minimizing potential risks.

- **First Trimester Meal Planning Tips**

Meal planning becomes essential during the first trimester of pregnancy since the mother's body undergoes major changes and the developing baby's nutritional needs increase. From the time of conception until week 12, there are a number of physiological changes that occur during this time, along with possible difficulties like exhaustion, morning sickness, and hormone changes. A healthy diet at this point provides a solid basis for the fetus's growth and development. Here are some crucial first-trimester meal planning suggestions to promote the health of the mother and feed the developing fetus.

Nutrient-Dense Foods: Prioritize nutrient-dense foods to meet increased nutritional demands. Lean proteins, complex carbohydrates, healthy fats, and a wide array of fruits and vegetables should constitute the core of your meals. This diverse range of nutrients aids in the baby's growth and supports the mother's overall well-being.

Folic Acid Intake: Folic acid is crucial in the early stages of pregnancy for neural tube development. Ensure adequate intake of foods rich in folate, such as leafy greens, lentils, citrus fruits, and fortified cereals. Your doctor might also recommend a folic acid supplement to meet the required dosage.

Hydration: Drink plenty of fluids, primarily water, throughout the day to stay hydrated. Dehydration can exacerbate pregnancy symptoms like fatigue and nausea. Herbal teas, fruit-infused water, and small amounts of natural juices can also contribute to hydration.

Frequent, Small Meals: Nausea and morning sickness are common during the first trimester. To combat these symptoms, opt for smaller, more frequent meals throughout the day rather than three large ones. This strategy helps maintain stable blood sugar levels and can alleviate nausea.

Mindful Eating: Listen to your body's cues and eat mindfully. Some women experience aversions or cravings during pregnancy. While it's essential to maintain a balanced diet, indulge in cravings in moderation and explore healthier alternatives when possible.

Include Iron-Rich Foods: Iron requirements increase during pregnancy to support the production of red blood cells. Incorporate iron-rich foods like lean meats, beans, lentils, spinach, and fortified cereals. Pairing these with foods high in Vitamin C enhances iron absorption.

Limit Caffeine and Avoid Risky Foods: Limit caffeine intake as excessive amounts can affect fetal development. Also, steer clear of risky foods like raw or undercooked meats, unpasteurized dairy products, and certain fish high in mercury content to reduce the risk of foodborne illnesses.

Supplements and Prenatal Vitamins: Consult with your healthcare provider to determine if prenatal vitamins or specific supplements are necessary. These can bridge nutritional gaps and ensure adequate intake of essential nutrients like calcium, vitamin D, and omega-3 fatty acids.

Healthy Snacking: Keep healthy snacks readily available to combat hunger and prevent energy dips. Nuts, yogurt, whole-grain crackers, and fresh fruits make excellent options that provide sustained energy and essential nutrients.

Consult a Dietitian or Nutritionist: Every pregnancy is unique, and individual dietary needs may vary. Seeking advice from a qualified dietitian or nutritionist can offer personalized guidance and ensure you're meeting specific nutritional requirements based on your health and lifestyle.

Rest and Stress Management: Adequate rest and stress management are vital components of a healthy pregnancy. Prioritize sleep and incorporate relaxation techniques like prenatal yoga, meditation, or deep breathing exercises to reduce stress levels.

Remember, while meal planning and nutrition are critical during pregnancy, it's equally important to maintain a balanced and holistic approach to overall health. Seek regular prenatal care, listen to your body, and communicate openly with your healthcare provider for guidance and support throughout this transformative journey.

Taking proactive steps to prioritize nutrition and overall well-being during the first trimester sets the stage for a healthier pregnancy, positively impacting both maternal and fetal health. By implementing these meal planning tips and making informed dietary choices, you can navigate the initial stages of pregnancy with confidence and support optimal development for you and your baby.

Recipes for the First Trimester

- **Energizing Breakfasts**

The first trimester of pregnancy is often accompanied by fluctuating energy levels and morning sickness. It's crucial to nourish your body with nutritious and easily digestible meals, especially in the morning. These energizing breakfast recipes aim to provide essential nutrients while being gentle on the stomach, offering a balance of flavors and textures to combat morning sickness and boost your energy throughout the day.

- **Banana Oatmeal Pancakes**

Prep Time: 10 minutes | Cook Time: 15 minutes | Total Time: 25 minutes

Ingredients:

- 1 ripe banana, mashed
- 1 cup rolled oats
- 1 egg (or substitute with a flax egg for a vegan option)
- ½ teaspoon baking powder
- ¼ teaspoon ground cinnamon

- ¼ cup milk (dairy or plant-based)
- 1 tablespoon honey or maple syrup (optional)
- Fresh fruits, yogurt, or nuts for topping

Instructions:

1. In a bowl, combine the mashed banana, oats, egg, baking powder, cinnamon, and milk. Mix until well combined. Let the batter sit for a few minutes to thicken.
2. Heat a non-stick pan over medium heat. Lightly grease the pan with cooking spray or a bit of oil.
3. Pour a small amount of batter onto the pan to form pancakes. Cook for 2-3 minutes until bubbles form on the surface, then flip and cook for an additional 1-2 minutes until golden brown.
4. Repeat until all the batter is used. Keep the cooked pancakes warm in a low-heated oven.
5. Serve the pancakes topped with fresh fruits, a dollop of yogurt, or a sprinkle of nuts. Drizzle with honey or maple syrup if desired.

- **Energizing Smoothie Bowl**

Prep Time: 10 minutes | Total Time: 10 minutes

Ingredients:

- 1 ripe banana, frozen
- 1 cup frozen mixed berries
- ½ cup spinach or kale leaves
- ½ cup Greek yogurt (or plant-based yogurt for a dairy-free option)
- ¼ cup almond milk or any preferred milk
- 1 tablespoon chia seeds or flaxseeds
- Toppings: sliced fruits, granola, shredded coconut, nuts, seeds, or honey

Instructions:

1. In a blender, combine the frozen banana, mixed berries, spinach or kale, yogurt, almond milk, and chia seeds. Blend until smooth and creamy.
2. Pour the smoothie into a bowl.
3. Arrange your desired toppings such as sliced fruits, granola, shredded coconut, nuts, seeds, or a drizzle of honey over the smoothie bowl.

- **Avocado Toast with Poached Egg**

Prep Time: 5 minutes | Cook Time: 5 minutes | Total Time: 10 minutes

Ingredients:

- 2 slices whole-grain bread
- 1 ripe avocado
- 2 eggs
- Salt and pepper to taste
- Optional toppings: cherry tomatoes, microgreens, or a sprinkle of red pepper flakes

Instructions:

1. Toast the slices of whole-grain bread to your desired level of crispness.
2. While the bread is toasting, scoop out the avocado flesh into a bowl and mash it with a fork. Season with salt and pepper.
3. Poach the eggs to your liking: bring a pot of water to a gentle simmer, add a splash of vinegar, crack the eggs into the water, and cook for about 3-4 minutes until the whites are set but the yolk is still runny.
4. Spread the mashed avocado onto the toasted bread slices.

5. Place a poached egg on each toast. Sprinkle with additional salt, pepper, and any optional toppings of your choice.

These energizing breakfast recipes are rich in essential nutrients, providing a balanced start to your day during the first trimester of pregnancy. They offer a blend of flavors and textures while being gentle on the stomach, helping you combat morning sickness and maintain your energy levels throughout the day.

- **Comforting Soups and Stews**

The first trimester of pregnancy is a critical time for both the mother and the developing fetus. During this period, many women experience morning sickness, nausea, and food aversions, making it challenging to maintain a balanced diet. However, it's crucial to consume nutritious meals to support the baby's growth and the mother's health. Comforting soups and stews can be a lifesaver during this phase, providing essential nutrients while being gentle on the stomach.

- **Ginger Carrot Soup**

Ingredients:

- 4 large carrots, peeled and chopped
- 1 onion, diced
- 2 cloves garlic, minced
- 1 tablespoon fresh ginger, grated
- 4 cups vegetable or chicken broth
- 1 tablespoon olive oil
- Salt and pepper to taste

Instructions:

1. Heat olive oil in a pot over medium heat. Add onions and garlic, sauté until translucent.
2. Add grated ginger and chopped carrots. Cook for 5 minutes, stirring occasionally.
3. Pour in the broth, bring to a boil, then reduce heat and simmer for 20-25 minutes until carrots are tender.
4. Using an immersion blender or regular blender, blend the soup until smooth.
5. Season with salt and pepper. Serve warm.

   Note: Ginger helps alleviate nausea, making this soup an excellent choice for easing morning sickness symptoms.

- **Chicken and Rice Congee**

Ingredients:

- 1 cup white rice
- 6 cups chicken broth
- 1 cup cooked chicken, shredded
- 1-inch piece ginger, thinly sliced
- 2 tablespoons soy sauce
- Sliced green onions for garnish
- Salt and pepper to taste

Instructions:

1. Rinse the rice under cold water until the water runs clear. In a large pot, bring the rice and chicken broth to a boil.
2. Reduce heat to low, add sliced ginger, and simmer, covered, for 40-45 minutes until the rice breaks down and the mixture thickens.
3. Stir occasionally to prevent sticking. Add shredded chicken and soy sauce, cook for an additional 10 minutes.
4. Season with salt and pepper. Serve hot, garnished with sliced green onions.

   Note: Congee is gentle on the stomach and provides comforting warmth, making it ideal for unsettled digestive systems.

- **Vegetable Lentil Stew**

Ingredients:

- 1 cup dried lentils, rinsed
- 4 cups vegetable broth
- 1 onion, diced
- 2 carrots, chopped
- 2 celery stalks, chopped
- 2 cloves garlic, minced
- 1 can diced tomatoes
- 1 teaspoon dried thyme
- 1 teaspoon paprika
- Salt and pepper to taste
- Olive oil for cooking

Instructions:

1. In a large pot, heat olive oil over medium heat. Add onions, carrots, and celery. Sauté until softened.
2. Add minced garlic, thyme, and paprika. Cook for an additional minute.
3. Stir in lentils, diced tomatoes, and vegetable broth. Bring to a boil, then reduce heat and simmer for 25-30 minutes until lentils are tender.
4. Season with salt and pepper. Serve piping hot.
   Note: Lentils are a great source of protein and iron, essential for the developing baby and the mother's energy levels.

- **Miso Soup with Tofu and Seaweed**

Ingredients:

- 4 cups water
- 4 tablespoons miso paste
- 1 cup tofu, cubed
- 2 tablespoons dried seaweed (wakame)
- 2 green onions, thinly sliced

Instructions:

1. In a pot, bring water to a simmer. Add dried seaweed and tofu cubes, cook for 2-3 minutes.
2. In a small bowl, dissolve miso paste in a ladleful of hot water from the pot.
3. Stir the miso paste mixture into the pot. Avoid boiling the soup after adding miso to preserve its nutrients.
4. Simmer for a few more minutes until heated through.
5. Garnish with sliced green onions and serve immediately.
   Note: Miso soup is rich in probiotics and provides a good source of protein and minerals, supporting a healthy pregnancy.

During the first trimester, staying hydrated and consuming easily digestible, nutrient-rich foods is crucial. These comforting soups and stews not only provide essential nutrients but also offer warmth and soothing relief for any pregnancy-related discomforts. Adjust spices and ingredients according to personal preferences and consult a healthcare professional for any specific dietary concerns during pregnancy.

- **Nourishing Snack Ideas**

During the first trimester of pregnancy, maintaining a well-balanced diet can be challenging due to nausea and food aversions. However, consuming nourishing snacks is essential to ensure both the mother's and baby's nutritional needs are met. Here are some delightful and easy-to-prepare snack ideas perfect for the first trimester.

- **Ginger Honey Lemon Tea**

Ingredients:

- 1-inch fresh ginger, thinly sliced
- 1 tablespoon honey
- Juice of 1 lemon
- 2 cups water

Instructions:

1. In a saucepan, bring water to a boil.
2. Add sliced ginger and let it simmer for 5-7 minutes.
3. Remove from heat, stir in honey and lemon juice.
4. Strain and serve warm. Ginger helps ease nausea, while lemon provides Vitamin C, and honey adds a touch of sweetness.

- **Avocado Toast with Whole Grain Bread**

Ingredients:

- 1 ripe avocado
- 2 slices whole grain bread
- Salt and pepper to taste
- Optional toppings: cherry tomatoes, sliced cucumber

Instructions:

1. Toast the bread slices until golden brown.

2. Mash the ripe avocado and spread it evenly on the toast.

3. Sprinkle it with salt and pepper.

4. Top with sliced cherry tomatoes or cucumber for added nutrients and flavor.

- **Yogurt Parfait with Berries and Nuts**

Ingredients:

- 1 cup Greek yogurt
- 1/2 cup mixed berries (strawberries, blueberries, raspberries)
- 2 tablespoons chopped nuts (almonds, walnuts)
- 1 tablespoon honey (optional)

Instructions:

1. In a bowl or glass, layer Greek yogurt, mixed berries, and chopped nuts.

2. Drizzle honey for sweetness if desired.

3. Repeat layers and enjoy this protein-rich and antioxidant-packed snack.

- **Baked Sweet Potato Chips**

Ingredients:

- 2 medium sweet potatoes
- 2 tablespoons olive oil
- 1 teaspoon paprika (optional)
- Salt to taste

Instructions:

1. Preheat the oven to 375°F (190°C) and line a baking sheet with parchment paper.

2. Wash and thinly slice the sweet potatoes.

3. In a bowl, toss the sweet potato slices with olive oil, paprika (if using), and salt.

4. Spread the slices in a single layer on the baking sheet.

5. Bake for 20-25 minutes or until crispy, flipping halfway through. These chips are a nutritious alternative to store-bought snacks.

- **Quinoa Salad Cups**

Ingredients:

- 1 cup cooked quinoa
- 1/2 cup diced cucumber
- 1/2 cup diced bell peppers (assorted colors)
- 1/4 cup chopped fresh parsley or cilantro
- 2 tablespoons olive oil
- 1 tablespoon lemon juice
- Salt and pepper to taste

Instructions:

1. In a bowl, mix cooked quinoa, diced cucumber, bell peppers, and chopped herbs.

2. Drizzle olive oil and lemon juice, season with salt and pepper, and toss until well combined.

3. Spoon the quinoa salad into lettuce cups for a refreshing and nutrient-packed snack.

- **Fruit Smoothie**

Ingredients:

- 1 ripe banana
- 1/2 cup frozen mixed berries
- 1/2 cup spinach or kale leaves
- 1 cup almond milk or yogurt
- 1 tablespoon chia seeds (optional)

1. Blend all ingredients until smooth and creamy.
2. Add more liquid if needed for desired consistency.
3. Chia seeds can be added for extra fiber and Omega-3 fatty acids.

These snacks offer a balance of essential nutrients crucial for the first trimester, combating nausea while providing energy and nourishment. Adjust ingredients according to personal preferences and dietary needs, ensuring a healthy and enjoyable snacking experience throughout this crucial stage of pregnancy.

- **Satisfying Main Courses**

During the first trimester of pregnancy, a woman's body goes through significant changes, often accompanied by morning sickness, fatigue, and various food aversions. It becomes crucial to focus on nutritious meals that are also gentle on the stomach. Here, we explore a selection of satisfying main course recipes designed to cater to the specific needs and cravings of expectant mothers during this stage.

- **Ginger-Lemon Chicken Soup**

Ingredients:

- 2 boneless, skinless chicken breasts
- 6 cups chicken broth
- 1 tablespoon grated fresh ginger
- 2 cloves garlic, minced

- 1 medium onion, finely chopped
- 2 carrots, sliced
- 1 celery stalk, diced
- Juice of 1 lemon
- Salt and pepper to taste
- Fresh parsley for garnish

Instructions:

1. In a large pot, bring chicken broth to a gentle boil.
2. Add chicken breasts to the pot and let them cook for 15-20 minutes until fully cooked. Remove the chicken and shred it using two forks.
3. In the same pot, add ginger, garlic, onion, carrots, and celery. Cook for 5-7 minutes until the vegetables are tender.
4. Return the shredded chicken to the pot and pour in lemon juice. Season with salt and pepper according to taste.
5. Let the soup simmer for an additional 10-15 minutes.
6. Garnish with fresh parsley before serving.

This comforting ginger-lemon chicken soup is rich in protein, vitamins, and minerals, offering a soothing remedy for queasiness while providing essential nutrients for both mother and baby.

- **Quinoa and Roasted Vegetable Salad**

Ingredients:

- 1 cup quinoa, rinsed
- 2 cups water or vegetable broth
- 1 red bell pepper, diced
- 1 yellow bell pepper, diced
- 1 small eggplant, diced

- 1 zucchini, diced
- 2 tablespoons olive oil
- 2 tablespoons balsamic vinegar
- 1 teaspoon dried thyme
- Salt and pepper to taste
- Fresh basil leaves for garnish

Instructions:

1. Preheat the oven to 400°F (200°C).
2. In a baking tray, toss the diced bell peppers, eggplant, zucchini with olive oil, balsamic vinegar, thyme, salt, and pepper.
3. Roast the vegetables for 20-25 minutes until they are tender and slightly browned.
4. Meanwhile, in a saucepan, combine quinoa and water or vegetable broth. Bring to a boil, then reduce heat, cover, and simmer for 15-20 minutes until the liquid is absorbed.
5. Once cooked, fluff the quinoa with a fork and let it cool slightly.
6. In a large bowl, mix the roasted vegetables with the cooked quinoa.
7. Garnish with fresh basil leaves before serving.

This quinoa and roasted vegetable salad provide a wholesome blend of fiber, vitamins, and antioxidants, aiding digestion and offering a colorful, flavorsome dish for expectant mothers.

- **Baked Salmon with Herbed Yogurt Sauce**

Ingredients:

- 4 salmon filets
- 1 tablespoon olive oil
- 2 teaspoons dried dill
- 1 teaspoon dried parsley
- 1 teaspoon garlic powder
- Salt and pepper to taste

Herbed Yogurt Sauce:

- 1 cup plain Greek yogurt
- 2 tablespoons fresh dill, finely chopped
- 1 tablespoon fresh parsley, finely chopped
- 1 tablespoon lemon juice
- 1 garlic clove, minced
- Salt and pepper to taste

Instructions:

1. Preheat the oven to 375°F (190°C).
2. Place the salmon filets on a baking sheet lined with parchment paper.
3. Drizzle olive oil over the salmon and sprinkle with dried dill, parsley, garlic powder, salt, and pepper.
4. Bake in the preheated oven for 12-15 minutes until the salmon is cooked through and flakes easily with a fork.
5. While the salmon is baking, prepare the herbed yogurt sauce by combining all the sauce ingredients in a bowl. Mix well and refrigerate until serving.
6. Serve the baked salmon with a dollop of herbed yogurt sauce on top.

Rich in omega-3 fatty acids and protein, baked salmon with herbed yogurt sauce offers a flavorful and nutritious option for expecting mothers, promoting the development of the baby's nervous system and providing essential nutrients.

These satisfying main course recipes aim to support the nutritional needs of expectant mothers during their first trimester while offering delicious and easily digestible options to ease common pregnancy-related discomforts.

- **Rejuvenating Beverages and Smoothies**

During the first trimester of pregnancy, when morning sickness might be at its peak, maintaining proper nutrition can be challenging. Rejuvenating beverages and smoothies can provide essential nutrients while soothing an unsettled stomach. Here are some recipes tailored to ease the queasiness and nourish the body during this critical phase of pregnancy:

- **Ginger Zest Smoothie**

Ingredients:

- 1 cup chopped fresh pineapple
- 1 ripe banana
- 1-inch piece of fresh ginger, peeled and chopped
- 1/2 cup Greek yogurt
- 1/2 cup coconut water or water
- Handful of ice cubes (optional)

Instructions:

1. Combine pineapple, banana, ginger, Greek yogurt, and coconut water in a blender.
2. Blend until smooth and creamy.
3. Add ice cubes if desired and blend again.
4. Pour into a glass and enjoy the refreshing and calming effects of ginger.

Ginger is known for its anti-nausea properties and can help alleviate morning sickness.

- **Berry Blast Energizer**

Ingredients:

- 1 cup mixed berries (strawberries, blueberries, raspberries)
- 1/2 cup spinach leaves (fresh or frozen)

- 1 tablespoon chia seeds
- 1/2 cup almond milk or any preferred milk
- 1/2 cup plain or vanilla yogurt
- Honey or maple syrup (optional for sweetness)

Instructions:

1. Combine mixed berries, spinach, chia seeds, almond milk, and yogurt in a blender.
2. Blend until the mixture reaches a smooth consistency.
3. Taste and add honey or maple syrup if desired for sweetness.
4. Pour into a glass and savor the nutritious mix of antioxidants, fiber, and vitamins.

The high antioxidant content of berries combined with spinach's iron and folic acid make this a powerhouse drink for expecting mothers.

- **Citrus Mint Refresher**

Ingredients:

- 2 oranges, peeled and segmented
- 1/2 cup chopped fresh pineapple
- 1/4 cup fresh mint leaves
- 1 tablespoon honey
- 1 cup coconut water or water
- Ice cubes (optional)

Instructions:

1. Place oranges, pineapple, mint leaves, honey, and coconut water in a blender.
2. Blend until the mixture is smooth.
3. Add ice cubes if desired and blend again.
4. Pour into a glass and relish the tangy, refreshing taste.

Citrus fruits are rich in vitamin C, while mint can aid digestion and soothe an upset stomach.

- **Green Protein Power Smoothie**

Ingredients:

- 1 ripe banana
- 1/2 ripe avocado
- 1 cup spinach leaves
- 1 tablespoon almond butter or peanut butter
- 1 scoop of plant-based protein powder (optional)
- 1 cup almond milk or any preferred milk

Instructions:

Combine banana, avocado, spinach, almond/peanut butter, protein powder (if using), and almond milk in a blender.
Blend until the mixture is creamy and well combined.
Pour into a glass and relish the nutrient-packed, creamy texture.

This smoothie is rich in potassium, healthy fats, and protein, providing an energy boost during the first trimester.

Tips:

- Small, Frequent Sips: Rather than drinking a large amount at once, take small sips throughout the day to manage nausea.
- Chill Ingredients: Using cold ingredients or adding ice can help ease the queasiness.
- Hydration: Remember to drink plenty of water between these rejuvenating beverages to stay hydrated.

These recipes are designed to be both nutritious and gentle on the stomach, aiming to alleviate morning sickness while providing essential nutrients crucial for the development of the baby. Adjust ingredients according to personal preferences and consult with a healthcare professional for personalized dietary advice during pregnancy.

Extra Tips and Advice

1. Coping with Morning Sickness

a. Eat Small, Frequent Meals: Consuming small, frequent meals throughout the day can help manage nausea. Avoid an empty stomach, as it can worsen symptoms.

b. Ginger and Peppermint: Ginger tea, ginger ale, or peppermint can help alleviate nausea. Some pregnant individuals find relief from morning sickness by sucking on peppermint candies or using ginger capsules.

c. Stay Hydrated: Dehydration can exacerbate nausea. Sip on water, clear broths, or electrolyte drinks to stay hydrated.

d. Acupressure Bands: Some women find relief from morning sickness by wearing acupressure bands, which target specific pressure points on the wrist.

e. Avoid Triggers: Certain smells, foods, or environments may trigger nausea. Identify and avoid these triggers whenever possible.

2. Handling Food Aversions and Cravings

a. Balanced Diet: Aim for a well-balanced diet even if certain foods are unappealing. Focus on incorporating other nutritious alternatives to ensure you're meeting your nutritional needs.

b. Experiment with Preparation: Try different cooking methods or recipes to make disliked foods more palatable. For example, if the taste or texture of a particular vegetable is off-putting, try steaming, roasting, or blending it into soups or smoothies.

c. Substitute Smartly: If you have an aversion to certain foods, find substitutes that provide similar nutritional benefits. For instance, if meat is unappealing, consider plant-based protein sources like tofu, lentils, or beans.

d. Indulge Cravings Wisely: While it's okay to indulge in cravings occasionally, try to do so in moderation. Opt for healthier versions or smaller portions to satisfy the craving without compromising on your overall nutrition.

3. Safe Exercise and Physical Activity

a. Consult Your Healthcare Provider: Before starting any exercise regimen, consult your healthcare provider to ensure it's safe for your pregnancy.

b. Low-Impact Activities: Opt for low-impact exercises like walking, swimming, prenatal yoga, or stationary cycling. These activities are generally safe and help maintain fitness without straining your body.

c. Avoid High-Risk Activities: Steer clear of activities with a high risk of falls or abdominal trauma. This includes contact sports, skiing, horseback riding, and activities that involve sudden movements or impacts.

d. Listen to Your Body: Pay attention to your body's signals. If you feel any discomfort, dizziness, or pain during exercise, stop immediately and consult your healthcare provider.

e. Stay Hydrated and Cool: Drink plenty of water before, during, and after exercise. Avoid overheating by exercising in well-ventilated areas and wearing loose, breathable clothing.

Remember, every pregnancy is unique, so what works for one person may not work for another. Prioritize your health and well-being by listening to your body and seeking guidance from healthcare professionals throughout your pregnancy journey.

Section 2

Second Trimester

- **Understanding the Second Trimester**

During pregnancy, the second trimester marks a remarkable phase characterized by several significant changes and milestones for both the expectant mother and the developing fetus. Lasting from week 13 to week 27, this trimester is often referred to as the "golden period" due to the easing of some initial pregnancy discomforts and the emergence of exciting developments.

Physical Changes

Maternal:

Growth and Glow: Many women experience a surge in energy and a sense of well-being during this phase. The infamous morning sickness tends to subside, and the "pregnancy glow" often becomes noticeable due to increased blood circulation and hormone levels.

Visible Changes: The baby bump becomes more pronounced as the uterus expands, leading to visible changes in the mother's body. The breasts continue to grow and prepare for lactation, and the skin might undergo changes due to hormonal fluctuations.

Movement Sensations: Around the midway point of the trimester, women typically start feeling the baby move, referred to as "quickening." These initial flutters gradually turn into more defined kicks and movements as the fetus grows.

Fetal:

Rapid Growth: The second trimester is a period of rapid growth for the fetus. Major organs and systems develop further, and by the end of this trimester, the baby's survival outside the womb significantly increases.

Sensory Development: Senses like hearing and sight begin to develop. The baby can hear sounds from the external environment and may even respond to voices or music.

Gender Identification: In most cases, the baby's gender becomes identifiable through ultrasound scans performed during this trimester.

Medical Check-ups and Tests

Regular prenatal check-ups are crucial during the second trimester to monitor the health and progress of both the mother and the baby. Some common tests and screenings during this phase include:

Ultrasound Scans: These scans offer detailed images of the fetus, helping doctors assess growth, development, and potential abnormalities.

Multiple Marker Screening: Usually performed between weeks 15 and 20, this blood test screens for genetic disorders such as Down syndrome and neural tube defects.

Glucose Screening: Around week 24 to 28, a glucose screening test is conducted to check for gestational diabetes.

Emotional and Psychological Changes

The relief from early pregnancy symptoms often brings a sense of emotional stability and joy during the second trimester. However, it's also a time when some women might experience heightened emotions or anxiety related to the impending changes and responsibilities.

Lifestyle Considerations

Nutrition: A well-balanced diet rich in nutrients is crucial for the health of both the mother and the developing baby. Iron, calcium, folic acid, and protein intake are particularly important.

Exercise: Moderate physical activity is encouraged unless otherwise advised by a healthcare provider. Prenatal yoga or swimming can help alleviate discomfort and improve overall well-being.

Rest and Sleep: As the pregnancy progresses, finding a comfortable sleeping position might become challenging. Adequate rest and sleep are essential, so experimenting with pillows or different sleeping arrangements can be beneficial.

In conclusion, the second trimester is a time of excitement, as the pregnancy becomes more tangible with the baby's movements and visible changes in the mother's body. It's crucial to maintain regular medical check-ups, adopt a healthy lifestyle, and address any concerns promptly to ensure a smooth and healthy pregnancy journey for both the mother and the growing baby.

- **Nutrition Guidelines for the Second Trimester**

During the second trimester of pregnancy, which spans from weeks 14 to 27, your body undergoes significant changes as your baby continues to grow and develop. Proper nutrition during this period is crucial to support your health and the healthy development of your baby. Here are comprehensive guidelines for nutrition during the second trimester:

Caloric Intake:
Your caloric needs may increase slightly during the second trimester, but it's important to focus on the quality of calories rather than just quantity. Aim for nutrient-dense foods to support your increased energy needs.

Protein:
Protein is essential for the growth of your baby's tissues and organs. Include lean meats, poultry, fish, eggs, dairy, legumes, and nuts in your diet. These sources provide essential amino acids necessary for fetal development.

Calcium:
Your baby's bones and teeth are forming, so ensure adequate calcium intake. Dairy products, fortified plant-based milks, tofu, broccoli, and leafy greens like kale and spinach are excellent sources of calcium.

Iron:
Iron is crucial for the increased blood supply and proper oxygen transport for both you and your baby. Include iron-rich foods like lean red meats, poultry, fish, beans, lentils, fortified cereals, and dark leafy greens. Pairing these with vitamin C-rich foods can enhance iron absorption.

Folate and Folic Acid:
Folate plays a vital role in preventing neural tube defects. Consume foods rich in folate, such as leafy greens, citrus fruits, legumes, fortified cereals, and supplements as recommended by your healthcare provider.

Omega-3 Fatty Acids:
These are essential for brain and vision development in the baby. Consume fatty fish (like salmon and sardines), flaxseeds, chia seeds, walnuts, and algae-based supplements to ensure an adequate intake.

Fiber:
Constipation is common during pregnancy. Increase fiber intake through whole grains, fruits, vegetables, legumes, and adequate hydration to prevent constipation and promote digestive health.

Hydration:
Drink plenty of water throughout the day. Staying hydrated helps support the increased blood volume, aids digestion, and helps prevent urinary tract infections.
Limit Caffeine and Avoid Alcohol: Limit caffeine intake to 200 mg per day or less (equivalent to about one 12-ounce cup of coffee). Avoid alcohol completely, as it can harm the baby's development.

Supplements:
Continue taking prenatal vitamins as recommended by your healthcare provider to ensure you're getting essential nutrients like iron, calcium, vitamin D, and others necessary for a healthy pregnancy.

Healthy Snacking:
 Opt for nutritious snacks like fruits, yogurt, nuts, whole-grain crackers with cheese, or vegetable sticks with hummus to keep energy levels stable between meals.

Food Safety:
 Avoid raw or undercooked meats, unpasteurized dairy products, certain fish high in mercury (like shark or swordfish), and deli meats to minimize the risk of foodborne illnesses.

Always consult with your healthcare provider or a registered dietitian to personalize your nutrition plan according to your specific needs and any potential complications during your pregnancy. Each woman's nutritional needs can vary, so individualized guidance is important for a healthy pregnancy during the second trimester.

- **Growth and Development Milestones**

Certainly! During the second trimester of pregnancy, which spans from week 13 to week 27, a significant transformation occurs in the development of the fetus. This period is often referred to as the "honeymoon phase" of pregnancy due to various factors, including reduced nausea for many expectant mothers and the visible growth of the baby bump. In this section, we'll delve into the growth and developmental milestones that characterize this crucial stage.

Physical Development:

Fetal Growth:

- *Size and Weight:* By the end of the second trimester, the fetus typically grows from around 3-4 inches in length to about 14-16 inches and gains significant weight, increasing from a few ounces to around 1.5 to 2.5 pounds.
- *Proportional Changes:* The baby's body starts to elongate, with limbs becoming more defined and proportionate. Facial features become distinct, including the eyes, nose, and ears. The skeleton, initially cartilaginous, begins to harden into bone.
- *Vernix Caseosa and Lanugo:* A protective covering called vernix caseosa develops on the baby's skin to shield it from the amniotic fluid. Lanugo, a fine layer of hair, covers the body to aid in temperature regulation.

Organ Development:

- *Organ Maturation:* Major organs such as the liver, kidneys, and lungs continue to mature and function. The baby's digestive system starts producing meconium, the earliest stool, while the lungs begin producing surfactant, a substance crucial for breathing after birth.

Sensory Development:

- *Sensory Abilities:* By the midpoint of the trimester, the fetus begins to respond to sound. It can hear the mother's voice and external noises, fostering auditory development. Taste buds form, and the baby starts to swallow and process amniotic fluid, potentially influencing future taste preferences.

Cognitive and Behavioral Development:

Movement:

- *Active Movement:* The fetus becomes more active, with increased limb movements and somersaults. These movements might be felt by the mother as "quickening," a sensation akin to fluttering or gentle kicks.

Reflexes:

- Sucking Reflex: The baby starts practicing sucking motions, a reflex essential for nursing after birth. Thumb sucking may even occur in the womb.
- *Grasping Reflex:* The baby's fingers can clasp and unclasp in response to stimuli, indicating the presence of the grasping reflex.

Emotional and Psychological Development:

Responsive Behavior:

- *Sensitivity to Stimuli:* While the exact emotional development is challenging to ascertain, research suggests that the fetus might react to stimuli, potentially indicating emotional responsiveness.

Maternal Changes:

Physical Changes:

- *Baby Bump:* The uterus expands significantly, becoming more noticeable as the pregnancy progresses. The mother's body undergoes changes to accommodate the growing fetus.
- *Energy Levels:* For many expectant mothers, the second trimester is characterized by increased energy levels and a reduction in early pregnancy symptoms such as nausea and fatigue.

Emotional Well-being:

- *Bonding:* As the baby's movements become more pronounced, mothers often experience a deeper emotional connection, fostering bonding before birth.
- *Anticipation and Preparation:* Expectant parents often begin preparations for the baby's arrival during this trimester, including setting up the nursery, attending prenatal classes, and making birth plans.

The second trimester serves as a pivotal phase in pregnancy, marking significant growth and developmental milestones for both the fetus and the expectant mother. It is a time of increasing excitement and anticipation as the pregnancy progresses towards the final trimester.

- **Iron-Rich Foods for Blood Support**

During the second trimester of pregnancy, which spans from weeks 14 to 27, your body and the developing baby undergo significant changes. One crucial aspect of this stage is the need for increased nutrients to support both your health and the baby's growth. Iron, in particular, plays a vital role as it helps in the production of hemoglobin, the protein in red blood cells that carries oxygen to tissues.

Pregnancy increases the demand for iron, as your body is tasked with producing more blood to support the growing baby and placenta. This is essential to prevent iron deficiency anemia, a condition that can lead to fatigue, weakness, and complications during pregnancy.

Incorporating iron-rich foods into your diet becomes even more important in the second trimester. Here are some excellent sources of iron to consider:

Lean Meats: Beef, pork, and poultry are rich in heme iron, the type of iron that is more easily absorbed by the body. Ensure meats are cooked thoroughly to avoid any risks of foodborne illnesses.

Fish: Certain fish like salmon, tuna, and sardines are not only high in iron but also provide omega-3 fatty acids, which are beneficial for both brain and eye development in the baby.

Beans and Legumes: Lentils, chickpeas, kidney beans, and black beans are great plant-based sources of iron. They also contain fiber and protein, providing additional nutritional benefits.

Leafy Green Vegetables: Spinach, kale, and Swiss chard are packed with iron. Pairing these veggies with vitamin C-rich foods can enhance iron absorption.

Fortified Cereals and Grains: Many breakfast cereals and grains are fortified with iron. Check the labels to identify those with added iron for an extra boost.

Nuts and Seeds: Pumpkin seeds, cashews, and almonds are not only tasty snacks but also contain iron. Additionally, they offer healthy fats and other essential nutrients.

Dried Fruits: Prunes, raisins, and apricots are convenient sources of iron. They can be added to cereals, yogurt, or eaten as a snack.

Remember, while these foods are rich in iron, your body's ability to absorb iron can be influenced by other dietary components. Pairing iron-rich foods with sources of vitamin C, like citrus fruits, tomatoes, or bell peppers, can enhance iron absorption.

However, it's essential to consult with your healthcare provider or a registered dietitian before making significant changes to your diet, especially during pregnancy. They can provide personalized recommendations based on your individual nutritional needs.

Maintaining adequate iron levels during pregnancy is crucial for both your well-being and the healthy development of your baby. Incorporating these iron-rich foods into your diet can help ensure you meet your body's increased demands during this important stage of pregnancy.

- **Second Trimester Meal Planning Strategies**

During the second trimester of pregnancy, which typically spans from weeks 13 to 27, many women find relief from the initial symptoms and discomforts experienced in the first trimester. This phase is often referred to as the "honeymoon period" of pregnancy due to increased energy levels and reduced nausea. However, it's still crucial to maintain a nutritious diet to support both the mother's health and the growing baby's development.

Meal planning during the second trimester should focus on providing essential nutrients, managing increased energy levels, and catering to potential new cravings or aversions. Here are some strategies and guidelines to consider:

Balanced Nutrition:

- *Protein Intake:* Ensure sufficient protein from sources like lean meats, poultry, fish, legumes, tofu, and nuts. Protein is vital for fetal development and helps in repairing tissues.
- *Calcium-Rich Foods:* Incorporate dairy products, fortified plant-based milk, leafy greens, and calcium-fortified foods to support bone and teeth development in the baby.
- *Iron-Rich Foods:* Consume iron-rich foods such as lean meats, spinach, lentils, and fortified cereals to prevent anemia and support blood production.
- *Folate and Vitamin B:* Include foods like dark leafy greens, citrus fruits, nuts, and whole grains to aid in neural tube development.

Frequent, Small Meals:

- Opt for smaller, more frequent meals to manage increased energy levels and help alleviate common pregnancy discomforts like heartburn and indigestion.
- Keep healthy snacks readily available to avoid excessive hunger and make healthier choices.

Hydration:

- Drink plenty of water throughout the day to stay hydrated. Dehydration can exacerbate common pregnancy issues like constipation.

Address Cravings and Aversions:

- Be flexible with meal planning to accommodate changing food preferences or aversions. Incorporate healthier versions of preferred foods whenever possible.

Omega-3 Fatty Acids:

- Consume foods rich in omega-3 fatty acids, such as fatty fish (like salmon), flaxseeds, chia seeds, or walnuts, which support the baby's brain and eye development.

Meal Prepping:

- Consider batch cooking and meal prepping to ensure convenient access to nutritious meals and snacks. This can be especially helpful during busy days or when fatigue sets in.

Consultation with a Healthcare Professional:

- Always consult with a healthcare provider or a registered dietitian to tailor meal plans according to individual needs, especially if dealing with specific dietary restrictions or complications during pregnancy.

Sample Meal Plan:

- *Breakfast:* Whole-grain toast with avocado and eggs, a side of Greek yogurt, and a fruit smoothie.
- *Snack:* Nuts and dried fruits or a piece of fruit with cheese.
- *Lunch:* Grilled chicken or tofu salad with mixed greens, quinoa, and a variety of colorful vegetables.
- *Snack:* Hummus with carrot sticks or whole-grain crackers.
- *Dinner:* Baked salmon with steamed broccoli and sweet potatoes.
- *Snack (if needed):* Greek yogurt with berries or a small bowl of oatmeal.

Remember, the second trimester is a time to embrace the changes in your body and adjust your diet accordingly. Prioritize nutrient-dense foods, stay hydrated, and listen to your body's cues for optimal health during this crucial phase of pregnancy.

Recipes for the Second Trimester

- **Power-Packed Salads and Bowls**

During the second trimester of pregnancy, maintaining a well-balanced diet is essential for both the mother's health and the baby's development. Incorporating nutrient-dense ingredients into your meals can be both delicious and beneficial. Salads and bowls offer a versatile and satisfying way to combine various nutrients, flavors, and textures in a single dish. Here are some power-packed recipes tailored for the second trimester:

- **Quinoa and Roasted Vegetable Salad**

Ingredients:

- 1 cup quinoa, rinsed
- 2 cups water or vegetable broth
- 2 cups mixed vegetables (bell peppers, zucchini, cherry tomatoes, etc.), chopped
- 2 tablespoons olive oil
- 2 tablespoons balsamic vinegar
- 1 teaspoon dried herbs (rosemary, thyme, or Italian seasoning)
- Salt and pepper to taste
- 1/4 cup crumbled feta cheese (optional)
- Fresh parsley for garnish

Instructions:

1. Preheat the oven to 400°F (200°C).
2. Toss chopped vegetables in olive oil, balsamic vinegar, dried herbs, salt, and pepper.
3. Spread the vegetables on a baking sheet and roast for 20-25 minutes or until tender.
4. Meanwhile, rinse quinoa and cook it in water or vegetable broth according to package instructions.
5. Once cooked, fluff the quinoa with a fork and let it cool slightly.
6. In a large bowl, combine quinoa and roasted vegetables. Toss gently.

7. Sprinkle with crumbled feta cheese (if using) and garnish with fresh parsley before serving.

- **Rainbow Buddha Bowl**

Ingredients:

- 1 cup cooked brown rice or quinoa
- 1 cup chickpeas, drained and rinsed
- 2 cups mixed greens (spinach, kale, arugula, etc.)
- 1/2 cup shredded purple cabbage
- 1 medium carrot, grated
- 1 ripe avocado, sliced
- 1/4 cup hummus
- Sesame seeds for garnish
- Dressing of choice (such as tahini-lemon or balsamic vinaigrette)

Instructions:

1. Arrange cooked rice or quinoa as the base in a bowl.
2. Divide and place chickpeas, mixed greens, shredded cabbage, grated carrot, and sliced avocado in sections over the base.
3. Dollop hummus in the center or in a separate section of the bowl.
4. Sprinkle sesame seeds over the bowl for added crunch and nutrition.
5. Drizzle with your preferred dressing or serve it on the side.

- **Mango, Avocado, and Black Bean Salad**

Ingredients:

- 2 ripe mangoes, peeled and diced
- 1 ripe avocado, diced
- 1 can (15 oz) black beans, drained and rinsed
- 1 red bell pepper, diced
- 1/4 cup red onion, finely chopped
- 1/4 cup fresh cilantro, chopped
- Juice of 1 lime
- 2 tablespoons olive oil
- Salt and pepper to taste

Instructions:

1. In a large bowl, combine diced mangoes, avocado, black beans, bell pepper, red onion, and cilantro.
2. In a small bowl, whisk together lime juice, olive oil, salt, and pepper to make the dressing.
3. Drizzle the dressing over the salad and toss gently to coat all ingredients evenly.
4. Allow the flavors to meld by refrigerating the salad for about 15-20 minutes before serving.

These power-packed salads and bowls not only offer a colorful array of nutrients but also provide ample fiber, vitamins, minerals, and healthy fats essential for a healthy pregnancy. Enjoy these recipes as part of a balanced diet to support your well-being during this crucial phase.

- **Wholesome Pasta and Grain Dishes**

Recipe 1: Roasted Vegetable Pasta

Ingredients:

- 1 medium eggplant, diced
- 1 zucchini, sliced
- 1 red bell pepper, chopped
- 1 yellow bell pepper, chopped
- 1 onion, thinly sliced
- 3 cloves garlic, minced
- 2 tablespoons olive oil
- Salt and pepper to taste
- 12 oz (340g) whole grain pasta
- 1 cup cherry tomatoes, halved
- ¼ cup fresh basil, chopped
- Grated Parmesan cheese (optional)

Instructions:

1. Preheat the oven to 400°F (200°C).
2. Place the diced eggplant, sliced zucchini, chopped bell peppers, sliced onion, and minced garlic on a baking sheet. Drizzle with olive oil, season with salt and pepper, and toss to coat.
3. Roast the vegetables in the preheated oven for 20-25 minutes or until they're tender and slightly caramelized.
4. Meanwhile, cook the pasta according to package instructions until al dente. Drain and set aside.
5. In a large bowl, combine the roasted vegetables, cooked pasta, cherry tomatoes, and fresh basil. Toss gently to mix.
6. Serve the pasta topped with grated Parmesan cheese if desired.

Recipe 2: Quinoa Stuffed Bell Peppers

Ingredients:

- 4 large bell peppers, any color
- 1 cup quinoa, rinsed
- 1 ¾ cups vegetable broth or water
- 1 can (15 oz) black beans, drained and rinsed
- 1 cup corn kernels (fresh or frozen)
- 1 can (14 oz) diced tomatoes, drained
- 1 teaspoon cumin
- 1 teaspoon chili powder
- Salt and pepper to taste
- ½ cup shredded cheddar cheese (optional)
- Chopped fresh cilantro for garnish

Instructions:

1. Preheat the oven to 375°F (190°C). Cut the tops off the bell peppers, remove seeds and membranes, and set aside.
2. In a saucepan, bring the vegetable broth or water to a boil. Add quinoa, reduce heat to low, cover, and simmer for 15-20 minutes or until the quinoa is cooked and liquid is absorbed.
3. In a large bowl, combine the cooked quinoa, black beans, corn, diced tomatoes, cumin, chili powder, salt, and pepper.
4. Stuff the bell peppers with the quinoa mixture and place them in a baking dish. If using cheese, sprinkle it over the stuffed peppers.
5. Cover the baking dish with foil and bake for 25-30 minutes until the peppers are tender.
6. Remove the foil and bake for an additional 5 minutes until the cheese is melted and bubbly.
7. Garnish with chopped cilantro before serving.

Recipe 3: Lemon Garlic Herb Orzo

Ingredients:

- 1 cup orzo pasta
- 2 tablespoons olive oil
- 3 cloves garlic, minced
- Zest of 1 lemon
- Juice of 1 lemon
- 2 tablespoons fresh parsley, chopped
- 1 tablespoon fresh thyme leaves
- Salt and pepper to taste
- Grated Parmesan cheese for serving (optional)

Instructions:

1. Cook the orzo according to package instructions. Drain and set aside.
2. Heat olive oil in a skillet over medium heat. Add minced garlic and cook for 1-2 minutes until fragrant but not browned.
3. Add cooked orzo to the skillet along with lemon zest, lemon juice, parsley, and thyme. Toss to combine and coat the orzo with the herbs and lemon.
4. Season with salt and pepper to taste.
5. Serve the lemon garlic herb orzo with grated Parmesan cheese on top if desired.

Enjoy these nutritious and flavorful pasta and grain dishes during your second trimester! Adjust ingredients or consult with a healthcare professional if you have any dietary restrictions or concerns during pregnancy.

- **Healthy Desserts and Treats**

During the second trimester of pregnancy, your cravings might be in full swing, and having healthier dessert options can satisfy those sweet tooth urges while providing essential nutrients for you and your growing baby. Here are some delightful and nutritious dessert recipes to enjoy during this phase:

- **Berry Chia Seed Pudding**

Ingredients:

- 1/4 cup chia seeds
- 1 cup almond milk (or any preferred milk)
- 1 teaspoon vanilla extract
- 1 tablespoon honey or maple syrup
- Assorted berries (strawberries, blueberries, raspberries) for topping

Instructions:

1. In a bowl, mix chia seeds, almond milk, vanilla extract, and honey/maple syrup. Stir well.
2. Let the mixture sit for about 15 minutes, stirring occasionally to prevent clumping.
3. Once the chia seeds have absorbed the liquid and the mixture thickens to a pudding-like consistency, refrigerate it for at least 2 hours or overnight.
4. Serve chilled, topped with assorted fresh berries.

Nutritional Benefits: Chia seeds are high in omega-3 fatty acids, fiber, protein, and various micronutrients. Berries are rich in antioxidants, vitamins, and fiber, contributing to a healthy pregnancy diet.

- **Baked Apple Slices**

Ingredients:

- 2 apples (any sweet variety)
- 1 tablespoon melted coconut oil or butter
- 1 teaspoon cinnamon
- 1 tablespoon honey or maple syrup (optional)
- Nuts or granola (optional, for topping)

Instructions:

1. Preheat the oven to 350°F (175°C).
2. Core and slice the apples thinly (about 1/4 inch slices). Leave the skin on for added nutrients.
3. In a bowl, toss the apple slices with melted coconut oil/butter, cinnamon, and honey/maple syrup (if using), ensuring the slices are evenly coated.
4. Place the slices on a baking sheet lined with parchment paper.
5. Bake for 20-25 minutes or until the apples are tender and slightly caramelized.
6. Serve warm, optionally topped with nuts or granola for added crunch.

Nutritional Benefits: Apples are a great source of fiber, vitamins, and antioxidants. This simple recipe adds natural sweetness without excessive sugars, offering a guilt-free dessert option.

- **Avocado Chocolate Mousse**

Ingredients:

- 2 ripe avocados
- 1/4 cup cocoa powder
- 1/4 cup honey or maple syrup

- 1 teaspoon vanilla extract
- Pinch of salt
- Optional toppings: sliced fruits, shredded coconut, nuts

Instructions:

1. Scoop out the flesh of the avocados and place them in a blender or food processor.
2. Add cocoa powder, honey/maple syrup, vanilla extract, and a pinch of salt.
3. Blend until smooth and creamy, scraping down the sides as needed to ensure everything is well combined.
4. Transfer the mousse to serving bowls or glasses.
5. Chill in the refrigerator for at least 30 minutes before serving.
6. Top with sliced fruits, shredded coconut, nuts, or any desired toppings.

Nutritional Benefits: Avocado provides healthy fats, fiber, and various vitamins, while cocoa powder offers antioxidants and a chocolatey flavor without the added sugar often found in conventional desserts.

- **Greek Yogurt Parfait**

Ingredients:

- 1 cup Greek yogurt (plain or flavored)
- 1/2 cup mixed fresh or frozen fruits (berries, sliced bananas, mango chunks)
- 1/4 cup granola or crushed nuts
- Drizzle of honey or maple syrup (optional)

Instructions:

1. In a glass or bowl, layer Greek yogurt, mixed fruits, and granola/crushed nuts alternatively.

2. Repeat the layers until the glass or bowl is filled.

3. Drizzle honey or maple syrup on top for added sweetness if desired.

4. Serve immediately as a delightful parfait.

Nutritional Benefits: Greek yogurt is a great source of protein and calcium, while fruits and granola provide vitamins, fiber, and healthy carbohydrates, making this parfait a balanced and satisfying dessert option.

- **Banana-Oat Cookies**

Ingredients:

- 2 ripe bananas, mashed
- 1 cup rolled oats
- 1/4 cup chopped nuts (walnuts, almonds, or pecans)
- 1/4 cup raisins or dark chocolate chips (optional)
- 1 teaspoon vanilla extract
- 1/2 teaspoon cinnamon
- Pinch of salt

Instructions:

1. Preheat the oven to 350°F (175°C) and line a baking sheet with parchment paper.

2. In a bowl, combine mashed bananas, rolled oats, chopped nuts, raisins/chocolate chips (if using), vanilla extract, cinnamon, and a pinch of salt. Mix well.

3. Scoop spoonfuls of the mixture onto the prepared baking sheet, flattening each cookie slightly with a spoon or your fingers.

4. Bake for 15-18 minutes or until the cookies are golden brown around the edges.

5. Allow the cookies to cool on the baking sheet for a few minutes before transferring them to a wire rack to cool completely.

Nutritional Benefits: These cookies offer a natural sweetness from bananas and optional dried fruits or chocolate chips. Rolled oats provide fiber, while nuts add healthy fats and additional nutrients.

Enjoy these delicious and healthy dessert options during your second trimester to satisfy cravings while supporting your and your baby's nutritional needs. Remember to consult with your healthcare provider about your dietary choices during pregnancy for personalized advice.

- **Hydrating Infusions and Drinks**

Certainly! Staying hydrated during pregnancy, especially in the second trimester, is crucial for both the expecting mother's health and the baby's development. Incorporating hydrating infusions and drinks can make hydration enjoyable and add essential nutrients. Here are several recipes perfect for the second trimester:

- **Citrus Infused Water:**

Ingredients:

- 1 lemon, sliced
- 1 lime, sliced
- 1 orange, sliced
- 8-10 cups of water
- Fresh mint leaves (optional)

Instructions:

1. Wash the citrus fruits thoroughly and slice them.

2. Fill a pitcher with water and add the sliced fruits.

3. For extra flavor, add a few fresh mint leaves.

4. Refrigerate for at least an hour before serving.

- **Cucumber Mint Cooler:**

Ingredients:

- 1 cucumber, sliced
- 1/4 cup fresh mint leaves
- 1 lemon, juiced
- 4 cups cold water
- Ice cubes

Instructions:

1. Blend cucumber slices and mint leaves with lemon juice until smooth.
2. Strain the mixture to remove any pulp.
3. Mix the cucumber-mint juice with cold water.
4. Serve over ice cubes for a refreshing drink.

- **Ginger-Lemonade Infusion:**

Ingredients:

- 4 cups water
- 1-inch piece of ginger, peeled and sliced
- 1/2 cup freshly squeezed lemon juice
- Honey or agave syrup (to taste)

Instructions:

1. In a saucepan, bring the water and ginger slices to a gentle boil.
2. Simmer for 5-7 minutes, then remove from heat and let it cool.
3. Once cooled, strain out the ginger pieces.
4. Add freshly squeezed lemon juice and sweeten with honey or agave syrup.
5. Chill and serve over ice.

- **Berry Blast Hydration Drink:**

Ingredients:

- 1 cup mixed berries (strawberries, blueberries, raspberries)
- 4 cups cold water
- 1 tablespoon honey or maple syrup (optional)

Instructions:

1. Blend the mixed berries with a little water until smooth.
2. Strain the berry puree to remove seeds.
3. Mix the strained berry juice with cold water.
4. Sweeten with honey or maple syrup if desired.
5. Chill and serve with ice.

- **Coconut Water Refresher:**

Ingredients:

- 2 cups coconut water
- 1 cup pineapple juice

- 1/2 cup mango juice
- Squeeze of lime juice
- Ice cubes

Instructions:

1. Mix coconut water, pineapple juice, mango juice, and lime juice in a pitcher.
2. Stir well and refrigerate until chilled.
3. Serve over ice cubes for a tropical hydrating treat.

These hydrating infusions and drinks are not only delicious but also provide essential nutrients, vitamins, and hydration during the second trimester of pregnancy. Always consult with a healthcare professional regarding any dietary changes during pregnancy.

Extra Tips and Advice

- **Managing Heartburn and Indigestion**

Pregnancy often brings on heartburn and indigestion due to hormonal changes and the growing uterus putting pressure on the stomach. To manage these discomforts:

- *Eat Small, Frequent Meals:* Opt for smaller meals throughout the day to prevent overloading your digestive system.
- *Avoid Trigger Foods:* Steer clear of spicy, acidic, and fatty foods that can exacerbate heartburn.
- *Stay Upright After Eating:* Give your body time to digest by staying upright for at least an hour after meals.

- *Sleeping Position:* Elevating your upper body slightly while sleeping can help alleviate nighttime heartburn.
- *Consult Your Doctor:* If these measures aren't helping, talk to your healthcare provider about safe antacids or other remedies.

- **Maintaining a Balanced Diet**

A well-rounded diet is crucial for both you and your baby's health. Consider these tips:

- *Eat a Variety of Foods:* Aim for a colorful plate with fruits, vegetables, whole grains, lean proteins, and healthy fats.
- *Stay Hydrated:* Drink plenty of water throughout the day to support your body's changing needs.
- *Iron-Rich Foods:* Incorporate iron-rich foods like spinach, beans, and lean meats to prevent anemia.
- *Calcium Intake:* Ensure you get enough calcium for bone health. Dairy products, leafy greens, and fortified foods are good sources.
- *Consult a Dietitian:* If you're unsure about meeting nutritional needs, seek guidance from a professional to create a tailored plan.

- **Preparing for Labor and Delivery**

As the due date approaches, it's natural to feel a mix of excitement and nerves. Here's how to prepare:

- *Childbirth Classes:* Consider enrolling in childbirth education classes to learn about labor, breathing techniques, and pain management.
- *Create a Birth Plan:* Outline your preferences for labor, such as pain relief options, who you want present, and post-birth preferences.
- *Pack Your Hospital Bag:* Pack essentials like comfortable clothing, toiletries, important documents, and items for both you and the baby.

- *Stay Active:* Engage in gentle exercises or prenatal yoga to keep your body prepared and alleviate stress.
- *Mental Preparation:* Practice relaxation techniques, visualize a positive birth experience, and discuss any fears or concerns with your healthcare provider or a counselor.

Remember, each pregnancy is unique, so trust your instincts and stay in communication with your healthcare provider for personalized guidance throughout this journey.

Section 3

Third Trimester

Understanding the Third Trimester

The third trimester of pregnancy is a crucial and transformative period that typically spans from week 28 to week 40, marking the final phase before childbirth. This stage is characterized by significant growth and development in both the fetus and the expectant mother. Understanding the changes, challenges, and necessary precautions during this trimester is paramount for ensuring a healthy pregnancy and childbirth experience.

Fetal Development

Rapid Growth: During the third trimester, the fetus undergoes remarkable growth and maturation. Organs such as the lungs, brain, and liver continue to develop, while the baby gains weight and accumulates body fat necessary for temperature regulation after birth.
Movement and Positioning: As the baby grows larger, its movements might feel more pronounced to the mother. The fetus tends to settle into a head-down position in preparation for birth. However, some babies might remain in a breech (bottom-down) or transverse (sideways) position, potentially requiring intervention or specialized delivery techniques.
Sensory Development: The fetus's sensory organs, such as sight and hearing, continue to mature. By the third trimester, the baby can distinguish between light and dark and can respond to sound stimuli from the external environment.

Maternal Changes and Considerations

Physical Changes: Expectant mothers might experience various physical discomforts during the third trimester, including increased back pain, heartburn, difficulty sleeping, and swelling in the feet and ankles due to fluid retention. The growing uterus can also cause shortness of breath as it presses against the diaphragm.

Emotional Rollercoaster: Hormonal changes, coupled with the anticipation of childbirth, can lead to heightened emotional states. It's common for pregnant individuals to experience mood swings, anxiety, or increased stress during this phase.

Prenatal Care: Regular prenatal check-ups become even more crucial in the third trimester. Monitoring the baby's growth, assessing the mother's health, and preparing for labor and delivery are key focuses during these visits.

Preparing for Labor and Delivery

Braxton Hicks Contractions: Often referred to as "practice contractions," these irregular contractions might become more noticeable in the third trimester. They help prepare the uterus for labor but are typically less intense and sporadic than true labor contractions.

Childbirth Education: Many expectant parents opt for childbirth classes during the third trimester to learn about the labor process, pain management techniques, and birthing options. These classes can help ease anxiety and build confidence for labor and delivery.

Birth Plan and Hospital Bag: Developing a birth plan detailing preferences for labor and delivery and packing a hospital bag with essentials for both the mother and baby are important tasks in the third trimester.

Potential Complications and Warning Signs

Preterm Labor: Any signs of preterm labor, such as regular contractions before 37 weeks, vaginal bleeding, or fluid leakage, require immediate medical attention.

Gestational Diabetes and Hypertension: Some women develop gestational diabetes or pregnancy-induced hypertension in the third trimester, necessitating careful monitoring and management by healthcare providers.

Decreased Fetal Movements: A noticeable decrease in the baby's movements or kick counts might indicate potential issues and should prompt a visit to the healthcare provider for assessment.

In conclusion, the third trimester of pregnancy is a time of significant physical, emotional, and psychological changes for both the mother and the developing fetus. By staying informed, attending regular prenatal check-ups, maintaining a healthy lifestyle, and seeking medical attention when necessary, expectant parents can navigate this crucial phase with confidence, preparing for the imminent arrival of their new family member.

Nutrition Guidelines for the Third Trimester

The third trimester of pregnancy is a crucial period for both the mother and the developing fetus. During this time, the nutritional needs of the mother continue to evolve, aiming to support the baby's growth and development while preparing the mother's body for childbirth and postpartum recovery. Here are essential nutrition guidelines to follow during this stage:

Increased Caloric Intake:
- As the baby grows rapidly in the final trimester, an increase in caloric intake becomes essential. An additional 300-500 calories per day are recommended to meet the increased energy demands.
- Focus on nutrient-dense foods rather than empty calories to ensure adequate nutrition for both the mother and the baby.

Protein-Rich Foods:
- Protein plays a crucial role in fetal development and helps in the formation of the baby's tissues and organs. Aim for 70-100 grams of protein daily.
- Sources of high-quality protein include lean meats, poultry, fish, eggs, dairy products, legumes, nuts, and seeds.

Iron-Rich Foods:
- Iron is vital for red blood cell production and preventing anemia, which is common during pregnancy. Increase iron intake to around 27 milligrams per day.

- Consume iron-rich foods like lean red meat, poultry, fish, beans, lentils, spinach, and fortified cereals. Pairing these foods with sources of vitamin C can enhance iron absorption.

Calcium and Vitamin D:

- Calcium is essential for the baby's bone development, while vitamin D aids in its absorption. Aim for 1,000-1,300 milligrams of calcium daily.
- Good sources of calcium include dairy products, fortified plant-based milk, leafy greens, tofu, and sardines. Exposure to sunlight helps the body produce vitamin D.

Omega-3 Fatty Acids:

- Omega-3s, particularly DHA (docosahexaenoic acid), are crucial for the baby's brain and eye development. Aim for 200-300 milligrams of DHA daily.
- Incorporate fatty fish like salmon, mackerel, and sardines into your diet. Vegetarian sources include flaxseeds, chia seeds, walnuts, and algae-based supplements.

Fiber-Rich Foods:

- Constipation is common during pregnancy, and consuming fiber can help alleviate this issue. Aim for 25-30 grams of fiber daily.
- Increase intake of fruits, vegetables, whole grains, legumes, and nuts to ensure an adequate fiber intake.

Hydration:

- Staying hydrated is crucial, especially during pregnancy. Aim to drink around 10-12 cups (2.4-3 liters) of fluids per day.
- Water is the best choice, but herbal teas, coconut water, and natural fruit juices (in moderation) can contribute to overall fluid intake.

Small, Frequent Meals:

- As the baby grows and takes up more space, consuming smaller, more frequent meals can help manage heartburn, indigestion, and discomfort.
- Opt for nutrient-dense snacks like yogurt, fruits, nuts, and whole-grain crackers between meals to maintain steady energy levels.

Be Mindful of Food Safety:

- Avoid certain foods like unpasteurized dairy, raw seafood, deli meats, and undercooked meats to reduce the risk of foodborne illnesses.
- Wash fruits and vegetables thoroughly, practice proper food handling and storage, and ensure meat is cooked to the recommended temperature.

Consultation with Healthcare Provider:

- Always consult your healthcare provider or a registered dietitian for personalized nutrition advice and guidance throughout your pregnancy journey.

By following these nutrition guidelines, expectant mothers can ensure optimal health for themselves and their developing babies during the crucial third trimester of pregnancy. Prioritizing a well-balanced diet, adequate hydration, and consulting healthcare professionals are key aspects of a healthy pregnancy journey.

☐ Final Preparations for Birth and Beyond

The third trimester, spanning from week 28 until birth, is an exciting and often physically demanding time for expectant parents. It's a period marked by a culmination of preparations for the imminent arrival of the baby and the final stages of pregnancy. Here's an extensive guide to Section 3: Third Trimester - Final Preparations for Birth and Beyond:

Physical Changes:

1. Weight Gain and Body Changes:

- *Increased Weight:* Most women will gain the most weight in this trimester, with the baby growing rapidly.
- *Bodily Changes:* The abdomen continues to expand, causing discomfort and changes in posture. Stretch marks and skin pigmentation might also become more prominent.

2. Discomforts:

- *Braxton Hicks Contractions:* These practice contractions become more frequent and intense.
- *Backaches and Joint Pains:* The extra weight puts pressure on the back and joints, leading to discomfort.
- *Shortness of Breath:* As the uterus expands, it can press against the diaphragm, making it harder to breathe.
- *Frequent Urination:* The growing uterus puts pressure on the bladder, causing more trips to the bathroom.

3. Fetal Development:

- *Baby's Growth:* The baby continues to gain weight and develop organs, including the brain, lungs, and immune system.
- *Baby's Movement:* Movements become more pronounced as the baby has less space to move around.

Health and Prenatal Care:

1. Prenatal Appointments:

- *Frequent Check-ups:* Visits to the obstetrician become more frequent, usually biweekly or even weekly in the last month.
- *Monitoring Baby's Health:* Tests like ultrasounds and non-stress tests may be performed to monitor the baby's health and position.

2. Diet and Exercise:

- *Healthy Eating:* A balanced diet rich in nutrients is crucial for both the baby's development and the mother's health.
- *Safe Exercise:* Gentle exercises like walking, prenatal yoga, and swimming can help with discomfort and prepare the body for labor.

3. Common Concerns:

- *Gestational Diabetes:* Screening tests are done to monitor blood sugar levels.
- *Preeclampsia:* Monitoring blood pressure and other symptoms is important to detect this condition.

Preparation for Birth:

1. Birth Plan:

- *Discussing Birth Preferences:* Parents-to-be should communicate their preferences for labor, delivery, and postpartum care with healthcare providers.

2. Childbirth Classes:

- *Educational Classes:* Attending childbirth classes can help prepare parents for labor, delivery, and caring for a newborn.

3. Nesting and Preparing for the Baby:

- *Setting Up Nursery:* Getting the baby's room ready with essentials like a crib, changing table, and baby clothes.
- *Packing Hospital Bag:* Preparing a bag with essentials for labor, delivery, and the hospital stay.

Emotional and Mental Preparation:

1. Anticipation and Anxiety:

- *Mixed Emotions:* Excitement, anxiety, and nervousness are common as the due date approaches.
- *Support System:* Building a support network and discussing fears and concerns with a partner or loved ones can help alleviate anxiety.

2. Bonding with Baby:

- *Prenatal Bonding:* Talking, singing, and spending quiet moments focusing on the baby can strengthen the bond before birth.

3. Self-Care:

- *Rest and Relaxation:* Getting adequate rest and practicing relaxation techniques can help manage stress.
- *Mindfulness and Mental Health*: Engaging in activities that promote mental well-being, such as meditation or prenatal massages, can be beneficial.

Final Preparations:

1. Legal and Practical Matters:

- *Birth Registration:* Understanding the process of birth registration and necessary documentation.
- *Maternity Leave and Work Arrangements:* Finalizing work arrangements and preparing for maternity or paternity leave.

2. Postpartum Planning:

- *Postpartum Support:* Discussing plans for postpartum support, such as help with household chores or hiring a doula.

3. Reviewing Birth Plans:

- *Revisiting Birth Preferences:* Going over the birth plan with the healthcare provider and making any necessary adjustments.

Conclusion:

The third trimester is a whirlwind of physical, emotional, and practical preparations as parents eagerly await the arrival of their baby. It's a time of nesting, bonding, and ensuring that everything is in place for the birth and the transition into parenthood. Taking care of one's physical and mental well-being while finalizing preparations is crucial for a smooth transition into the next chapter of life.

- **Calcium-Rich Foods for Bone Development**

During the third trimester of pregnancy, the development of the baby's bones and skeletal system becomes a prominent focus. Calcium plays a crucial role in ensuring the proper formation and strength of the baby's bones, teeth, and overall skeletal structure. As such, incorporating calcium-rich foods into the mother's diet during this stage is essential to support the growing needs of both the mother and the developing fetus.

Here are some calcium-rich foods that can be beneficial for bone development during the third trimester:

Dairy Products:
- Milk, yogurt, and cheese are excellent sources of calcium. They also provide other essential nutrients like protein, vitamins, and minerals necessary for both the mother and the baby's growth.

Leafy Green Vegetables:
- Dark, leafy greens such as kale, spinach, collard greens, and broccoli are rich in calcium. These vegetables also contain other nutrients like vitamin K, which supports bone health by aiding in calcium absorption.

Fortified Foods:

- Many food products, such as certain cereals, bread, and juices, are fortified with calcium. These can be beneficial sources of calcium, especially for individuals who might not consume dairy or other traditional sources of this mineral.

Tofu and Soy Products:

- Tofu made with calcium sulfate and some soy products are good non-dairy sources of calcium. Incorporating these into the diet can provide a plant-based alternative for obtaining calcium.

Nuts and Seeds:

- Almonds, chia seeds, sesame seeds, and certain nuts like Brazil nuts and almonds contain calcium. These can be included as snacks or added to meals to boost calcium intake.

Fish with Edible Bones:

- Some fish, such as canned salmon or sardines, are consumed with their bones and provide a significant amount of calcium. These can be part of a balanced diet to contribute to the required calcium intake.

Legumes and Beans:

- Certain legumes like chickpeas, lentils, and beans (such as black beans, kidney beans) contain moderate amounts of calcium. They also offer fiber and protein, making them valuable additions to a pregnancy diet.

Fortified Plant-Based Milk Alternatives:

- Options like fortified almond milk, soy milk, or oat milk can provide a calcium boost for those who prefer plant-based or lactose-free alternatives to dairy.

It's important to note that along with calcium, other nutrients such as vitamin D, magnesium, phosphorus, and vitamin K are also crucial for optimal bone health. Vitamin D, for instance, aids in the absorption of calcium in the body. Therefore, ensuring a well-balanced diet that includes these nutrients along with regular prenatal vitamins recommended by healthcare providers is crucial for supporting bone development during the third trimester of pregnancy.

- **Third Trimester Meal Planning Techniques**

Congratulations! You've reached the third trimester of your pregnancy, an exciting time as you prepare for the arrival of your little one. During this phase, proper nutrition is crucial for both you and your growing baby. Meal planning becomes even more essential to ensure you're meeting your nutritional needs while managing any discomforts that may arise during this period.

- **Focus on Nutrient-Rich Foods**

In the third trimester, your baby is rapidly developing and gaining weight. It's important to consume nutrient-dense foods to support their growth and development. Prioritize the following nutrients:

a. Protein

- *Sources:* Lean meats, poultry, fish, eggs, legumes, nuts, and seeds.
- *Importance:* Supports the baby's tissue growth and helps in the development of organs.

b. Calcium

- *Sources:* Dairy products, fortified plant-based milk, leafy greens (such as kale, spinach), and tofu.
- *Importance:* Aids in the development of your baby's bones and teeth.

c. Iron

- *Sources:* Red meat, poultry, fish, lentils, beans, fortified cereals.
- *Importance:* Helps in the production of red blood cells to prevent anemia.

d. Omega-3 Fatty Acids

- *Sources:* Fatty fish (salmon, mackerel), chia seeds, flaxseeds, walnuts.
- *Importance:* Supports brain and eye development in the baby.

e. Folate/Folic Acid

- *Sources:* Leafy greens, citrus fruits, beans, fortified grains.
- *Importance:* Reduces the risk of neural tube defects in the baby.

- **Plan Small, Frequent Meals**

As your baby grows, your stomach has less space, making it uncomfortable to eat large meals. Opt for smaller, more frequent meals throughout the day to manage heartburn, indigestion, and bloating. This approach also helps maintain steady energy levels.

- **Stay Hydrated**

Drink plenty of water throughout the day to stay hydrated. Dehydration can lead to complications such as urinary tract infections and premature contractions. Aim for at least 8-10 glasses of water daily.

- **Prepare for Quick and Easy Meals**

In the final trimester, fatigue might increase, making it challenging to cook elaborate meals. Prepare and freeze meals in advance, or stock up on easy-to-prepare items like pre-cut vegetables, frozen fruits, whole-grain pasta, and canned beans for quick, nutritious meals.

- **Incorporate Snacks**

Healthy snacks can help curb hunger between meals and provide essential nutrients. Consider snacks like yogurt with fruit, whole-grain crackers with nut butter, vegetable sticks with hummus, or a handful of nuts and dried fruits.

- **Consider Supplements**

Consult your healthcare provider about continuing prenatal vitamins. They might recommend additional supplements such as calcium or iron based on your individual needs.

- **Be Mindful of Food Safety**

Avoid foods that pose a risk of foodborne illnesses, such as unpasteurized dairy, undercooked meat, raw fish, and certain types of deli meats. Properly handle and cook foods to prevent foodborne illnesses that could harm you and your baby.

Conclusion

The third trimester is a critical time for both you and your baby. By focusing on nutrient-rich foods, staying hydrated, planning small meals, and being mindful of food safety, you can support your health and the healthy development of your baby. Always consult your healthcare provider or a registered dietitian for personalized guidance and recommendations during this special phase of your pregnancy.

Recipes for the Third Trimester

1. Nutrient-Dense Smoothie Bowls

Green Goddess Smoothie Bowl

Ingredients:

- 1 ripe banana, frozen
- 1 cup spinach leaves
- 1/2 cup kale leaves, stems removed
- 1/2 cup unsweetened almond milk
- 1 tablespoon chia seeds
- 1 tablespoon almond butter
- Toppings: Sliced fruits, granola, shredded coconut

Instructions:

1. In a blender, combine the frozen banana, spinach, kale, almond milk, chia seeds, and almond butter. Blend until smooth.
2. Pour the smoothie into a bowl and arrange your favorite toppings on top.
3. Enjoy this nutrient-packed bowl for a refreshing and filling meal.

2. Comforting One-Pot Meals

Vegetable Quinoa Stew

Ingredients:

- 1 cup quinoa, rinsed
- 2 cups vegetable broth
- 1 tablespoon olive oil

- 1 onion, chopped
- 2 cloves garlic, minced
- 2 carrots, diced
- 2 celery stalks, chopped
- 1 bell pepper, diced
- 1 can (15 oz) diced tomatoes
- 1 teaspoon dried thyme
- Salt and pepper to taste
- Fresh parsley for garnish

Instructions:

1. In a large pot, heat olive oil over medium heat. Add onions and garlic, sauté until fragrant.
2. Add carrots, celery, and bell pepper. Cook for a few minutes until slightly softened.
3. Stir in diced tomatoes, quinoa, vegetable broth, thyme, salt, and pepper. Bring to a boil, then reduce heat and let it simmer for 15-20 minutes until quinoa is cooked and vegetables are tender.
4. Adjust seasoning if needed. Serve hot, garnished with fresh parsley.

3. Energy-Boosting Snacks

Almond Butter Energy Balls

Ingredients:

- 1 cup rolled oats
- 1/2 cup almond butter
- 1/4 cup honey or maple syrup
- 1/4 cup chopped nuts (walnuts, almonds, or cashews)
- 1/4 cup shredded coconut
- 1 teaspoon vanilla extract
- Pinch of salt

Instructions:

1. In a bowl, mix together rolled oats, almond butter, honey/maple syrup, chopped nuts, shredded coconut, vanilla extract, and a pinch of salt.
2. Roll the mixture into small balls using your hands.
3. Place the energy balls on a baking sheet lined with parchment paper and refrigerate for at least 30 minutes to set.
4. Enjoy these energy-boosting snacks whenever you need a quick bite.

4. Soothing Herbal Teas and Elixirs

Ginger-Lemon Pregnancy Elixir

Ingredients:

- 2-inch piece of fresh ginger, thinly sliced
- 4 cups water
- Juice of 1-2 lemons
- Honey to taste

Instructions:

1. In a saucepan, bring water to a boil. Add sliced ginger and let it simmer for 10-15 minutes.
2. Remove from heat and strain the ginger-infused water into a mug.
3. Add fresh lemon juice and honey to taste. Stir well.
4. Sip on this soothing elixir to ease digestion and provide a refreshing boost.

These recipes aim to provide essential nutrients, comfort, and energy for the third trimester of pregnancy. Always consult with a healthcare professional for personalized dietary advice during pregnancy.

Extra Tips and Advice

1. Dealing with Swelling and Discomfort

a. Hydration and Nutrition:

- Drink plenty of water to stay hydrated and reduce fluid retention.
- Consume foods rich in potassium (bananas, sweet potatoes) to help regulate fluid balance.

b. Elevation and Rest:

- Elevate swollen body parts, especially feet and ankles, when sitting or lying down.
- Take regular breaks to rest and elevate legs above the heart level to reduce swelling.

c. Compression and Massage:

- Use compression stockings or sleeves to alleviate swelling in the legs.
- Gentle massages can help improve circulation and reduce discomfort.

d. Comfortable Clothing and Footwear:

- Wear loose, comfortable clothing to allow better blood flow.
- Opt for supportive, low-heeled shoes to minimize foot and ankle swelling.

e. Cold Compresses:

- Apply cold compresses or ice packs (wrapped in a cloth) to swollen areas for short intervals to reduce inflammation.

f. Consultation with Healthcare Provider:

- If swelling is sudden or severe, or if accompanied by symptoms like headaches or visual disturbances, seek immediate medical attention.

2. Preparing for Breastfeeding

a. Attend Prenatal Classes:

- Consider attending breastfeeding classes to learn proper techniques and address concerns.

b. Invest in Proper Gear:

- Purchase comfortable nursing bras and tops that provide easy access for breastfeeding.
- Consider a breast pump to express milk if needed.

c. Establish Support Networks:

- Seek guidance from lactation consultants, friends, or family members experienced in breastfeeding.
- Join local or online support groups for breastfeeding mothers.

d. Educate Yourself:

- Learn about the benefits of breastfeeding for both mother and baby.
- Understand common challenges and how to overcome them, such as latching difficulties or engorgement.

e. Practice Relaxation Techniques:

- Stress can affect milk production. Practice relaxation techniques like deep breathing or meditation to promote a calm environment for breastfeeding.

f. Be Patient and Persistent:

- Breastfeeding might take time to establish. Be patient with yourself and your baby, and don't hesitate to ask for help if needed.

3. Creating a Relaxing Birth Environment

a. Birth Plan Preparation:

- Create a birth plan that outlines your preferences for the birthing environment, pain management, and support during labor.

b. Comfort Measures:

- Pack comfort items such as music playlists, essential oils, or a favorite pillow to create a familiar and soothing atmosphere.
- Consider using birthing balls, water therapy, or massage techniques for pain relief.

c. Communication with Birth Team:

- Communicate your preferences and needs clearly with your birth team (medical professionals, midwives, or doulas) to create a supportive environment.

d. Visualization and Relaxation Techniques:

- Practice visualization or guided imagery exercises to promote relaxation during contractions.

e. Flexible Mindset:

- Stay open-minded as labor progresses. Birth plans might need adjustments, and flexibility can reduce stress.

f. Partner or Support Person Involvement:

- Encourage your partner or chosen support person to actively participate in creating a calming environment and providing emotional support.

Remember, every pregnancy and birth experience is unique. Prioritize self-care, gather knowledge, and communicate openly with healthcare providers to ensure a smooth transition into motherhood.

Section 4

Postpartum and Beyond

- **Postpartum Nutrition and Recovery**

Postpartum nutrition is crucial for aiding recovery and supporting the body after childbirth. During this phase, focus on nourishing foods rich in nutrients that aid healing and replenish depleted stores. Iron-rich foods like lean meats, beans, and leafy greens can help combat postpartum fatigue caused by blood loss during childbirth. Foods high in omega-3 fatty acids, such as salmon and flaxseeds, can assist in reducing inflammation and supporting brain health, which is important for both the mother and the baby.

Hydration is also essential, especially if breastfeeding. Drinking plenty of water and consuming fluids like herbal teas can aid in milk production and help the body recover from childbirth. It's important to include a variety of foods in your diet to ensure you're getting all the necessary vitamins and minerals to support your body during this time.

- **Breastfeeding Diet Essentials**

For breastfeeding mothers, maintaining a healthy diet is key to producing nutritious breast milk. Consuming a balanced diet that includes a variety of fruits, vegetables, whole grains, lean proteins, and healthy fats is important. Foods rich in calcium, such as dairy products, leafy greens, and fortified foods, can help maintain strong bones and support the baby's growth.

Avoiding excessive caffeine, alcohol, and certain medications that may pass into breast milk is recommended. Some babies may react negatively to certain foods consumed by their mothers, so paying attention to any reactions in the baby after feeding can help identify potential allergens.

- **Quick and Healthy Meals for New Moms**

New moms often face time constraints, making it challenging to prepare elaborate meals. Opting for quick and nutritious meals is essential during this phase. Meal prepping can be a lifesaver—prepare large batches of healthy meals and snacks in advance to have them readily available when time is limited.

Consider meals that are easy to assemble, such as salads with pre-cut veggies, grilled chicken or tofu, and a variety of dressings or sauces for flavor. Overnight oats or smoothie packs made with fruits, vegetables, and protein sources like Greek yogurt or protein powder can serve as quick and nourishing breakfast options. Snacks like nuts, fruits, cheese, and whole-grain crackers can provide energy and nutrients in between meals.

- **Introducing Solids to Your Baby**

Around six months of age, most babies are ready to start trying solid foods alongside breast milk or formula. Start with single-ingredient, pureed or mashed foods like avocado, banana, sweet potatoes, or steamed carrots. Gradually introduce new foods, waiting a few days between each new item to watch for any allergic reactions.

As your baby grows, offer a variety of textures and flavors to expand their palate and provide a range of nutrients. Avoid honey and foods that can be choking hazards, such as whole grapes or chunks of hard food. Continue breastfeeding or providing formula as the primary source of nutrition while introducing solids as a complement to their diet.

- **Continuing Healthy Eating Habits**

Beyond the postpartum period, maintaining healthy eating habits is essential for both the mother and the child. Incorporating a balanced diet rich in fruits, vegetables, whole grains, lean proteins, and healthy fats supports overall health and well-being.

Meal planning and preparation remain beneficial to ensure access to nutritious meals despite a busy schedule. Involving the family in mealtime and exposing children to a variety of healthy foods can help instill good eating habits from an early age.

Regular exercise, adequate sleep, and managing stress are also crucial components of postpartum and ongoing health. Remember to consult with healthcare professionals for personalized guidance on nutrition and well-being during the postpartum period and beyond.

Recipes for Postpartum and Beyond

Bringing a new life into the world is a joyous experience, but it also requires immense care and attention, especially in the postpartum period. Nutrition plays a crucial role during this time, aiding in recovery and providing essential nutrients for both the mother and the newborn. Here are a variety of recipes tailored for postpartum mothers and babies, ensuring convenience, nutrition, and ease of preparation.

- **Quick and Nutritious Breakfast Ideas**

a. Overnight Oats with Berries and Nuts

Ingredients:

- 1 cup rolled oats
- 1 cup milk (almond, soy, or regular)
- ½ cup Greek yogurt
- 1 tablespoon honey or maple syrup
- Fresh berries (strawberries, blueberries)
- Chopped nuts (almonds, walnuts)
- 1 teaspoon chia seeds (optional)

Instructions:

1. Mix oats, milk, yogurt, and sweetener in a jar or bowl.
2. Cover and refrigerate overnight.
3. In the morning, top with fresh berries, nuts, and chia seeds for added nutrition.
4. Enjoy!

b. Avocado Toast with Poached Egg

Ingredients:

- 2 slices whole-grain bread
- 1 ripe avocado
- 2 eggs
- Salt and pepper to taste
- Optional: cherry tomatoes, microgreens

Instructions:

1. Toast the bread slices.
2. Mash the avocado and spread it on the toast.
3. Poach the eggs to desired consistency.

4. Place poached eggs on the avocado toast.
5. Season with salt and pepper.
6. Serve with cherry tomatoes and microgreens if desired.

- **Easy-to-Prepare Lunches and Dinners**

a. Quinoa and Veggie Stir-Fry

Ingredients:

- 1 cup quinoa
- 2 cups vegetable broth or water
- Assorted vegetables (bell peppers, broccoli, carrots)
- 2 tablespoons olive oil
- 2 cloves garlic, minced
- Soy sauce or tamari to taste
- Optional: cooked chicken or tofu for added protein

Instructions:

1. Rinse quinoa and cook it in vegetable broth or water according to package instructions.
2. Heat olive oil in a pan, add minced garlic, and sauté for a minute.
3. Add chopped vegetables and cook until tender yet crisp.
4. Stir in cooked quinoa and soy sauce.
5. Add cooked chicken or tofu if desired.
6. Serve hot.

b. One-Pot Lentil Soup

Ingredients:

- 1 cup dried lentils, rinsed
- 1 onion, chopped
- 2 carrots, diced
- 2 celery stalks, diced
- 4 cups vegetable or chicken broth
- 1 can diced tomatoes
- 2 cloves garlic, minced
- 1 teaspoon cumin
- Salt and pepper to taste
- Fresh parsley for garnish

Instructions:

1. In a large pot, sauté onions, carrots, and celery until softened.

2. Add minced garlic and cumin, cook for another minute.
3. Add lentils, diced tomatoes, and broth.
4. Bring to a boil, then reduce heat and simmer for 20-25 minutes until lentils are tender.
5. Season with salt and pepper.
6. Garnish with fresh parsley before serving.

- **Snacks for New Moms and Babies**

a. Fruit and Nut Energy Balls

Ingredients:

- 1 cup dates, pitted
- 1 cup nuts (almonds, cashews)
- ¼ cup dried fruits (raisins, apricots)
- 2 tablespoons chia seeds
- 2 tablespoons honey
- Shredded coconut (optional)

Instructions:

1. In a food processor, blend dates, nuts, dried fruits, chia seeds, and honey until a sticky mixture forms.
2. Roll the mixture into small balls.
3. Optional: Roll the balls in shredded coconut for added flavor.
4. Refrigerate and enjoy as a quick energy boost.

b. Apple Slices with Nut Butter

Ingredients:

- 2 apples, sliced
- Nut butter (almond, peanut)
- Optional: honey or cinnamon for drizzling

Instructions:

1. Slice the apples into wedges.
2. Spread nut butter on each slice.
3. Drizzle with honey or sprinkle cinnamon for extra taste.
4. Serve immediately.

- **Homemade Baby Food Recipes**

a. Sweet Potato and Carrot Mash

Ingredients:

- 1 sweet potato, peeled and diced
- 2 carrots, peeled and chopped
- Water or vegetable broth

Instructions:

1. Steam or boil sweet potato and carrots until tender.
2. Blend or mash the cooked vegetables together.
3. Add water or vegetable broth as needed for desired consistency.
4. Cool and serve to your baby.

b. Banana and Avocado Puree

Ingredients:

- 1 ripe banana
- 1 ripe avocado

Instructions:

1. Mash the banana and avocado together until smooth.
2. Add breast milk or formula for desired consistency.
3. Serve immediately or refrigerate for later use.

These recipes are designed to provide nourishment, convenience, and variety for new mothers and their babies during the crucial postpartum period and beyond. Prioritize nutrition, rest, and self-care to support your health and well-being during this special time.

Extra Tips and Advice

Self-Care for New Moms

Prioritize Rest: Lack of sleep is common for new moms. Try to rest whenever the baby sleeps, even if it means leaving chores undone. Your well-being is crucial for both you and your baby.

Accept Help: Don't hesitate to ask for assistance from your partner, family, or friends. Whether it's help with household chores, preparing meals, or watching the baby for a short while, accepting support can ease the load.

Nourish Yourself: Eating well is essential for postpartum recovery. Focus on balanced meals that include protein, healthy fats, fruits, and vegetables. Consider meals that can be prepared in advance to save time.

Stay Hydrated: Drinking enough water is crucial, especially if you're breastfeeding. Keep a water bottle handy to ensure you're getting an adequate amount of fluids throughout the day.

Find Moments for Yourself: Carve out time for activities you enjoy. Whether it's reading, taking a walk, or simply having a quiet moment, self-care contributes to your mental well-being.

Connect with Other Moms: Joining mom groups or forums can provide support, advice, and a sense of community. Sharing experiences with others going through similar situations can be incredibly comforting.

Consider Professional Support: If feelings of sadness, anxiety, or overwhelming stress persist, seek guidance from a mental health professional. Postpartum depression is common and treatable, and it's important to prioritize your mental health.

Bonding Activities with Your Baby

Skin-to-Skin Contact: Holding your baby against your skin can promote bonding, regulate their temperature, and soothe them. This practice can be done during feeding times or simply for comfort.

Eye Contact and Talking: Engaging in eye contact and talking to your baby helps in building a strong emotional connection. Babies are responsive to voices and facial expressions.

Massage and Gentle Touch: Gently massaging your baby or using light touch can be calming and strengthen the bond between you and your little one.

Reading and Singing: Reading books or singing songs to your baby, even if they're too young to understand, helps in forming a routine and creates a comforting environment.

Baby-Wearing: Using a baby carrier allows for close physical contact while keeping your hands free. This practice can soothe your baby and help them feel secure while allowing you to move around more freely.

Play and Exploration: As your baby grows, engaging in age-appropriate play and exploration activities fosters bonding and encourages their development.

Long-Term Nutritional Guidelines

Balanced Diet: As your child grows, continue focusing on a balanced diet for yourself. Model healthy eating habits for your child by incorporating a variety of nutritious foods into your meals.

Include Whole Foods: Incorporate whole grains, lean proteins, fruits, and vegetables into your diet. These foods provide essential nutrients for both you and your child.

Stay Hydrated: Drinking water remains crucial. Encourage your child to develop healthy hydration habits by setting an example.

Limit Processed Foods and Sugars: Be mindful of the intake of processed foods and sugars in your family's diet. Instead, opt for homemade meals and snacks whenever possible.

Regular Meals and Snacks: Establishing regular meal times and healthy snack options can support your child's growth and development while maintaining good eating habits.

Consult a Pediatrician or Nutritionist: If you have specific concerns about your child's nutritional needs or dietary restrictions, seek guidance from a healthcare professional for personalized advice.

Remember, each mother-baby relationship is unique. Finding what works best for you and your baby may take time and adjustment. Prioritize your well-being while nurturing a loving and healthy bond with your little one.

Conclusion:

Throughout the exploration of the Pregnancy Cookbook by Trimester, we've delved into a comprehensive guide tailored to support expecting mothers through their incredible journey. Here's a recap of the key points highlighted in each trimester:

First Trimester: Nourishing Foundations

During the initial trimester, the emphasis was on establishing a strong foundation for both mother and baby. The focus was on combating morning sickness, providing essential nutrients for fetal development, and adapting to the changing dietary needs. The cookbook offered recipes rich in folate, iron, and other crucial vitamins and minerals necessary for the initial stages of pregnancy.

Second Trimester: Vital Growth and Energy

Moving into the second trimester, the cookbook provided recipes that catered to the increasing nutritional demands and energy requirements. The focus was on supporting the baby's rapid growth while also aiding the mother in maintaining her health and stamina. Emphasis was placed on calcium, protein, and omega-3 fatty acids to support bone development, muscle growth, and brain function.

Third Trimester: Preparation and Sustenance

The final trimester brought attention to preparation for childbirth and nourishing the body to support the baby's full-term growth. The recipes offered were aimed at boosting energy, aiding in digestion, and addressing common discomforts such as heartburn or swelling. Nutrient-dense meals were encouraged, particularly those containing protein, fiber, and healthy fats, to support the baby's development and aid the mother in preparation for labor.

Encouragement and Final Words:

Embarking on the journey of pregnancy is a remarkable and transformative experience, one filled with both joys and challenges. As you've engaged with this cookbook, may you have gained a deeper understanding of the crucial role nutrition plays in supporting both maternal and fetal health.

Remember, the journey of pregnancy is unique for each woman. It's essential to listen to your body, consult healthcare professionals, and embrace the changes occurring within you. This cookbook aimed to be a supportive companion, offering guidance and delicious recipes tailored to each stage of pregnancy.

As you prepare for the arrival of your little one, cherish these moments and the nourishment you provide, not just through meals but also through self-care and mindfulness. Embrace this special time, knowing that you are creating a nurturing environment for your baby's growth and development.

In closing, may this cookbook have empowered you with knowledge and recipes to support your well-being during this remarkable journey. Wishing you a smooth and healthy pregnancy, an empowering birth experience, and the joy of welcoming your bundle of joy into the world. Congratulations on this beautiful chapter of life!